AF340687

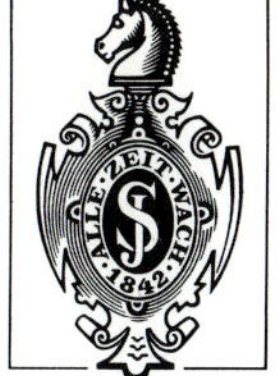

Sandostatin® in the Treatment of Acromegaly

Consensus Round Table, Amsterdam 1987

Editor: Steven W. J. Lamberts

With 78 Figures and 37 Tables

Springer-Verlag Berlin Heidelberg New York
London Paris Tokyo

Professor Steven W. J. Lamberts, M.D.
Rotterdam, University Hospital, Dijkzigt
Dr Molewaterplein 40
3015 GD Rotterdam
The Netherlands

ISBN 3-540-19269-7 Springer Verlag Berlin Heidelberg New York
ISBN 0-387-19269-7 Springer Verlag New York Berlin Heidelberg

Library of Congress Cataloging-in-Publication Data

Sandostatin® in the treatment of acromegaly.
1. Octreotide acetate−Therapeutic use−Testing−Congresses. 2. Acromegaly−Chemotherapy−
Congresses. I. Lamberts, Steven W. J. [DNLM: 1. Acromegaly−drug therapy−congresses.
2. Somatostatin−analogs & derivatives−congresses. 3. Somatostatin−therapeutic use−congresses.
WK 550 S218 1987]
RC658.3.S26   1988   616.4′7   88-17620
ISBN 0-387-19269-7 (U.S.)

Typesetting, printing and binding: Graphischer Betrieb K. Triltsch, Würzburg
2329/3321-543210 − Printed on acid-free paper

Table of Contents

Abbreviations

ACTH	adrenocorticotrophic hormone		NIDDM	non insulin-dependent diabetes mellitus
b.i.d.	bis in die (twice a day)		NMR	nuclear magnetic resonance
Br	bromocriptine		NTEL	no-toxic-effect level
CSF	cerebrospinal fluid		OD	oculus dexter (right eye)
CSI	continuous subcutaneous infusion		OGTT	oral glucose tolerance test
CT	computed tomography		OS	oculus sinister (left eye)
DA	dopamine		PET	positron emission tomography
FSH	follicle stimulating hormone		PIIIP	procollagen III propeptide
5-FU	5-fluorouracil		PRL	prolactin
GH	growth hormone		RER	rough endoplasmic reticulum
GHRH	growth hormone releasing hormone		RIA	radioimmunoassay
			RRA	radioreceptor assay
GnRH	gonadotropin releasing hormone		Sm-C	somatomedin-C
GRF	growth hormone releasing factor		SMS	Sandostatin
HPLC	high performance liquid chromatography		SRIF, SS	somatostatin (somatotropin release inhibiting factor)
IBMX	isobutylmethylxanthine		t.d.s.	ter die sumendum (to be taken three times a day)
IGF I	insulin-like growth factor I			
IRI	immunoreactive insulin		TFA	total fatty acids
LH	luteinizing hormone		t.i.d.	ter in die (three times a day)
LHRH	luteinizing hormone releasing hormone		TRH	thyrotropin releasing hormone
			T_3RU	triiodothyronine resin uptake
MRI	magnetic resonance imaging		TSH	thyroid stimulating hormone
mRNA	messenger ribonucleic acid			

Authors' Addresses

Baister, Elizabeth, B.Sc., MPS
Clinical Research Associate
Medical Department
Sandoz Pharmaceuticals
98, The Centre
Feltham, Middlesex TW13 4EP
(Great Britain)

Barkan, Ariel, M.D.
Asst Professor of Internal Medicine
University of Michigan
University Hospital
3920 Taubman Building
Ann Arbor, MI 48109 (USA)

Bayard, Francis, M.D.
Professor of Medicine
Head, Dept of Endocrinology
C.H.U. Rangueil
Université Paul Sabatier
Chemin du Vallon
31054 Toulouse Cedex (France)

Boerlin, Victor, M.D.
Head, Dept of Neuroendocrinology
Clinical Research
Sandoz Ltd
Pharma Division
4002 Basle (Switzerland)

Chiodini, Pier Giorgio, M.D.
Asst Endocrinologist
Divisione di Endocrinologia Carati
Ospedale Niguarda – Cà Granda
Piazza Ospedale Maggiore, 3
20162 Milan (Italy)

Deidier, Annick, M.D.
Project Leader
Clinical Research
Laboratoires Sandoz S.à.r.l.
51 rue Louis Blanc
69006 Lyon (France)

George, Susan R., M.D.,
F. R. C. P. (C), F. A. C. P.
Asst Professor, Attending Staff Physician
in Endocrinology
Eaton Wing 11N-227
Department of Medicine
Toronto General Hospital

University of Toronto
200 Elizabeth Street
Toronto, Ontario M5G 1C2 (Canada)

Ginsburg, Jean, M.D., D.M., F.R.C.P.
The Royal Free Hospital
London (Great Britain)

Harris, Alan G., M.D.
Medical Expert
Department of Neuroendocrinology
Clinical Research
Sandoz Ltd
Pharma Division
4002 Basle (Switzerland)

Imura, Hiroo, M.D.
Professor of Medicine
Second Department of Internal Medicine
Faculty of Medicine, Kyoto University
Seigoin Kawara-machi, Sakyo-ku
606 Kyoto (Japan)

Jackson, Ivor M.D., M.D.
Professor of Medicine, Physician in Charge
Department of Endocrinology
Brown University, Rhode Island Hospital
593 Eddy Street
Providence, Rhode Island 02903 (USA)

Kendall-Taylor, Pat, M.D., F.R.C.P.
Professor of Endocrinology
Department of Medicine
Royal Victoria Infirmary
Queen Victoria Road
NE1 4LP Newcastle upon Tyne
(Great Britain)

Killinger, Donald, M.D., M.Sc., Ph.D.,
F.R.C.P. (C)
Associate Professor
University of Toronto
Sr Staff Physician and Director
Clinical Investigation Unit
Wellesley Hospital
160 Wellesley St East
Toronto, Ontario M4Y 1J3 (Canada)

Lamberts, Steven W. J., M.D.
Professor of Internal Medicine
Rotterdam, University Hospital, Dijkzigt
Dr Molewaterplein 40
3015 GD Rotterdam (The Netherlands)

Landolt, Alex M., M.D.
Professor of Medicine
Asst Medical Director
Neurochirurgische Klinik
Universitätsspital Zürich
Rämistrasse 100
8091 Zurich (Switzerland)

Liuzzi, Antonio, M.D.
Asst Endocrinologist
Divisione di Endocrinologia Carati
Ospedale Niguarda – Cà Granda
Piazza Ospedale Maggiore, 3
20162 Milan (Italy)

de Longueville, Marc, M.D.
Clinical Research Monitor
Sandoz S.A.
Chaussée de Haecht 226
1030 Bruxelles (Belgium)

Marbach, Peter, M.D.
Preclinical Research
Sandoz Ltd
Pharma Division
4002 Basle (Switzerland)

Ørskov, Hans, M.D.
Professor of Medicine
Institute of Experimental Clinical Research
University of Aarhus
Kommunehospitalet
8000 Aarhus C (Denmark)

Pieters, Gerlach, M.D.
Radboud Hospital
University of Nijmegen
Geertgroteplein 8
Nijmegen (The Netherlands)

Plöckinger, Ursula, M.D.
Medizinische Klinik und Poliklinik
Universitätsklinikum Steglitz
der Freien Universität Berlin
Hindenburgdamm 30
1000 Berlin 45 (West Germany)

Quabbe, Hans-Jürgen, M.D.
Professor of Medicine
Medizinische Klinik und Poliklinik
Universitätsklinikum Steglitz
der Freien Universität Berlin
Hindenburgdamm 30
1000 Berlin 45 (West Germany)

Sassolas, Geneviève, M.D.
Hôpital Neuro-Cardiologique
Centre de Médecine Nucléaire
59 boulevard Pinel
69394 Lyon Cedex 3 (France)

Stevenaert, Achille, M.D.
Professor of Neurosurgery
Department of Neurosurgery
Hôpital de Bavière
Boulevard de la Constitution 66
4020 Liège (Belgium)

Thorner, Michael, M.B., F.R.C.P.
Professor of Medicine
Head, Division of Endocrinology
Department of Internal Medicine
University of Virginia, School of Medicine
Box 511
Charlottesville, Virginia 22908 (USA)

Vance, Mary Lou, M.D.
Asst Professor of Medicine
Department of Internal Medicine
University of Virginia, School of Medicine
Box 511
Charlottesville, Virginia 22908 (USA)

Wass, John A.H., M.D., F.R.C.P.
Reader in Medicine
and Consultant Physician
Department of Endocrinology
St Bartholomew's Medical School
West Smithfield
EC 1A 7BE London (Great Britain)

von Werder, Klaus, M.D.
Professor of Medicine
Asst Medical Director
Medizinische Klinik Innenstadt
der Universität München
Ziemssenstrasse 1
8000 München 2 (West Germany)

Nomenclature

Sandostatin®
Octreotide INN, BAN

Octréotide INN (F)
Octreotida INN (Span.)

1. Clinical Aspects of Growth Hormone Hypersecretory States

M. O. Thorner, M. L. Hartman, M. L. Vance

Division of Endocrinology, Department of Internal Medicine, University of Virginia, School of Medicine, Charlottesville, Virginia, USA

Growth hormone (GH) is secreted by the anterior pituitary and the pattern of secretion in both human and animal species is pulsatile [6, 19]. Thus, there are episodes of enhanced growth hormone secretion which occur at varying intervals. At present it is not clear whether growth hormone is tonically secreted between secretory bursts or whether it is only secreted episodically. Episodic growth hormone secretion is thought to be mediated by dual stimulation by hypothalamic growth hormone releasing hormone (GHRH) associated with a reduction in the tonic secretion of somatostatin (growth hormone release inhibiting hormone: SS) [18, 22]. Evidence from animal studies indicates that pulses of growth hormone secretion require GHRH, since passive immunization with antibodies to GHRH abolishes these GH bursts [24]. In contrast, basal growth hormone secretion is apparently tonically inhibited by somatostatin since passive immunization with antibodies to somatostatin leads to an increase in basal GH secretion [25]. The exact nature of hypothalamic secretion of somatostatin and GHRH is speculated to be reciprocal (Fig. 1) [18, 22]. This hypothesis has been supported by direct sampling of hypophyseal-portal blood in rats [12].

Growth hormone secretion is also regulated by peripheral factors which feed back at the hypothalamic and pituitary levels. Somatomedin-C (insulin-like growth factor I: IGF I) secretion is regulated by growth hormone when the nutritional state is adequate. IGF I feeds back at the pituitary and the hypothalamic level to inhibit growth hormone secretion. It is also likely that many other hormonal and metabolic factors feed back on growth hormone secretion and this has been extensively reviewed by Reichlin [13].

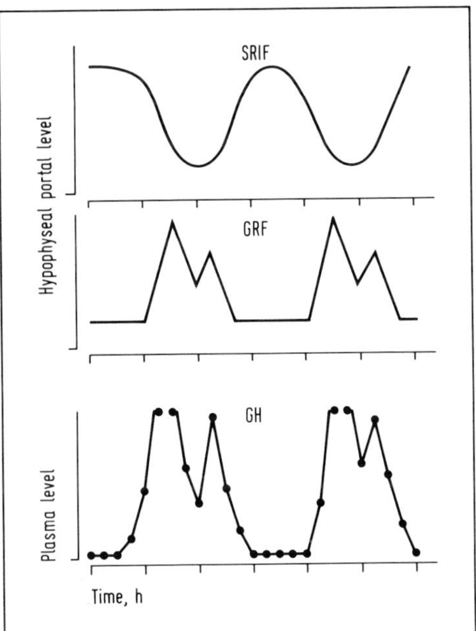

Fig. 1. Schematic representation of the postulated rhythmic secretion of SS and GHRH into hypophyseal-portal blood, with the net result on GH secretion, as observed in plasma. *SRIF* somatotropin release inhibiting factor, *GRF* growth hormone releasing factor, *GH* growth hormone. (Reproduced by permission from [18])

Growth Hormone Hypersecretory States

Growth hormone secretion is tightly regulated. The secretion of growth hormone varies with developmental stage, age, gonadal function, and sex. At birth growth hormone secretion is high, declines over the first few weeks of life, remains low throughout childhood, and increases at the time of puberty. Growth hormone secretion is greater in women than in men [6]. As individuals age growth hormone secretion is said to decline. Additionally, growth hormone secretion is enhanced in undernourished individuals [17], while in obese subjects growth hormone secretion is suppressed [26]. In a study which we performed several years ago, we examined the pulsatile secretion of growth hormone in normal adults who were categorized as young or older depending on age. Since all subjects were of normal weight, we were able to examine the effects of age, sex, and gonadal function on the pattern of growth hormone secretion. Using stepwise regression analysis, we observed that the single most important determinant of growth hormone secretion, characterized as area under the curve, amplitude of growth hormone pulses, or fraction of growth hormone secreted in pulses, was the circulating total free estradiol concentration [6]. The serum testosterone level did not correlate with these parameters of growth hormone secretion. We therefore believe that estradiol is very important in regulating growth hormone secretion in man.

Growth hormone hypersecretory states may, rarely, reflect either end organ resistance to growth hormone's actions, as in Laron dwarfism, or poor nutritional states such as are seen in protein-calorie malnutrition [17], or anorexia nervosa. However, the diagnosis of these states is usually obvious since the child either does not grow (in Laron dwarfism), or the appearance of a malnourished individual is clearly obvious. Similarly, in patients with diabetes mellitus, growth hormone secretion may be high but this is usually associated with normal or low somatomedin-C levels. In this meeting we are concerned with inappropriate hypersecretion of growth hormone which causes the clinical syndrome of acromegaly. In this situation growth hormone levels, in both the basal state and after ingestion of oral glucose, are high. Additionally, serum somatomedin-C levels are elevated. Thus, the patient who presents with symptoms and signs of acromegaly, who does not have diabetes mellitus, renal failure, or hepatic failure, who has high GH and somatome-

din-C levels, and lack of GH suppression to < 2 ng/ml after ingestion of oral glucose (e.g. 50 or 100 g) is, by definition, considered to have acromegaly.

The etiology of acromegaly is either hypothalamic, pituitary, or ectopic disease. Below we will discuss each, but it should be pointed out that more than 99 % of cases of acromegaly are a result of a primary pituitary tumor [20].

Occasionally acromegaly is a result of a gangliocytoma of the hypothalamus which secretes GHRH [2]. Neuronal tumors were described on one occasion as having grown down the pituitary stalk and having given rise to a pituitary tumor which surrounds the GHRH-secreting neurons. Since there are less than ten reported cases of this syndrome in the world literature, this must be considered an extremely unusual cause of acromegaly.

The most common cause of acromegaly is a pituitary tumor. In the past, the diagnosis of acromegaly was usually delayed by at least 15 years after the onset of symptoms of the condition. More recently, with an increased awareness of the symptoms, signs, and the ease of diagnosis, the disorder is detected much earlier. Thus, while previously most cases were often diagnosed in the fourth or fifth decades of life, now more cases are being diagnosed in the second and third decades. As discussed below, this should greatly improve the prognosis in such patients. The tumors may be solely growth hormone secreting, or may secrete both growth hormone and prolactin. Rarely, a tumor may secrete multiple anterior pituitary hormones including the glycoprotein hormones [9]. The classification is based not only on the patient's hormonal profile but, more recently, on the results of immunocytochemical studies of the tissue removed at operation.

Very rarely acromegaly is caused by peripheral tumors which secrete growth hormone releasing hormone [16, 21]. In this situation somatotroph hyperplasia occurs and careful morphologic examination of the pituitary tissue does not reveal a discrete pituitary tumor. The characteristics of somatotroph hyperplasia include: 1) intermingling of other pituitary cell types among a preponderance of somatotrophs; 2) retention of reticulin fibers within the pituitary so that the pituitary is still divided into acini; and 3) electron microscopic appearance of the somatotroph demonstrating stimulation of hormone synthesis and release indicated by well-developed Golgi apparatus and rough endoplasmic reticulum with the cells filled with secretory granules [21]. There have been between twenty and thirty cases in the world literature describing this syndrome. It should be noted that the isolation of the growth hormone releasing hormone was achieved from two tumors removed from patients with acromegaly secondary to ectopic GHRH secretion [5, 15, 16, 21].

The laboratory diagnosis of acromegaly will be discussed in the next chapter. However, in order to distinguish ectopic GHRH production as a cause of acromegaly it is necessary to measure the plasma GHRH level. Since ectopic GHRH secretion occurs in less than 1% of acromegalic patients, it might be argued that this investigation would be of low yield. However, for the patient who has ectopic GHRH as a cause of acromegaly it is important that this diagnosis be made prospectively. We have been involved with the prospective diagnosis of one such patient and this avoided unnecessary pituitary surgery.

The incidence and prevalence of acromegaly is difficult to assess and Christy and Warren report that in the USA 250 to 300 new cases are diagnosed annually [3]. The reported incidence and prevalence was 3 per million per year and 40 per million, respectively, in the Newcastle region of England [1]. In general, it is considered that tumors secreting ACTH giving rise to Cushing's disease are the most infrequent of the anterior pituitary tumors, and acromegaly or somatotroph adenomas are the second least common.

Clinical Symptoms and Signs

Patients with acromegaly have a gradual progression of symptoms and signs. It is for this reason that the diagnosis is often missed for many years. The symptoms usually begin insidiously and the changes in the body occur so slowly that the patient may not even notice them until complications develop (Fig. 2). The symptoms can be a result of the pituitary tumor itself, in which case the patient develops headaches and/or visual disturbances which may either be a visual field defect, or diplopia from external ophthalmoplegia. Hypopituitarism may occur if the tumor is very large; gonadal dysfunction is much more frequent than hypothyroidism and hypoadrenalism. More commonly, however, the patient presents with symptoms due to the effects of long-standing overproduction of growth hormone. If the patient develops the condition prior to puberty, there may be excessive growth, a condition which is termed gigantism. More commonly, the condition occurs after puberty and the patient develops enlargement of the hands and feet; rings become tighter, cannot be removed and may have to be cut off. The increased hand and finger size may cause difficulty with performing fine tasks such as picking up a pin from the floor. Glove size also increases. Similarly, shoe size increases, particularly the shoe width. Head size increases and for those who wear hats, there is an increase in hat size. Similarly, joint pain from accelerated osteoarthrosis may be the presenting symptom and may be misdiagnosed as "arthritis". The high levels of growth hormone are associated with excessive sweating and thus patients notice that they sweat more, particularly from the face, hands, and feet. Hyperhidrosis is sometimes the presenting symptom. Similarly, the increased soft tissues may lead to compression of the median nerve giving rise to carpal tunnel syndrome. The high growth hormone levels are diabetogenic and the patient may present with mild diabetes mellitus. Mild hypertension is also common. General organomegaly occurs and, in the late stages of the disease, a cardiomyopathy may occur giving rise to heart failure. The increased growth of the lower jaw causes prognathism and larger spaces between the teeth. The resultant malocclusion leads to temporomandibular arthritis. The tongue also becomes enlarged and may give rise to obstructive sleep apnea.

The increased soft tissue and bone mass is associated with an increased incidence of osteoarthrosis. This is particularly severe in the hips and knees, which results in considerable morbidity.

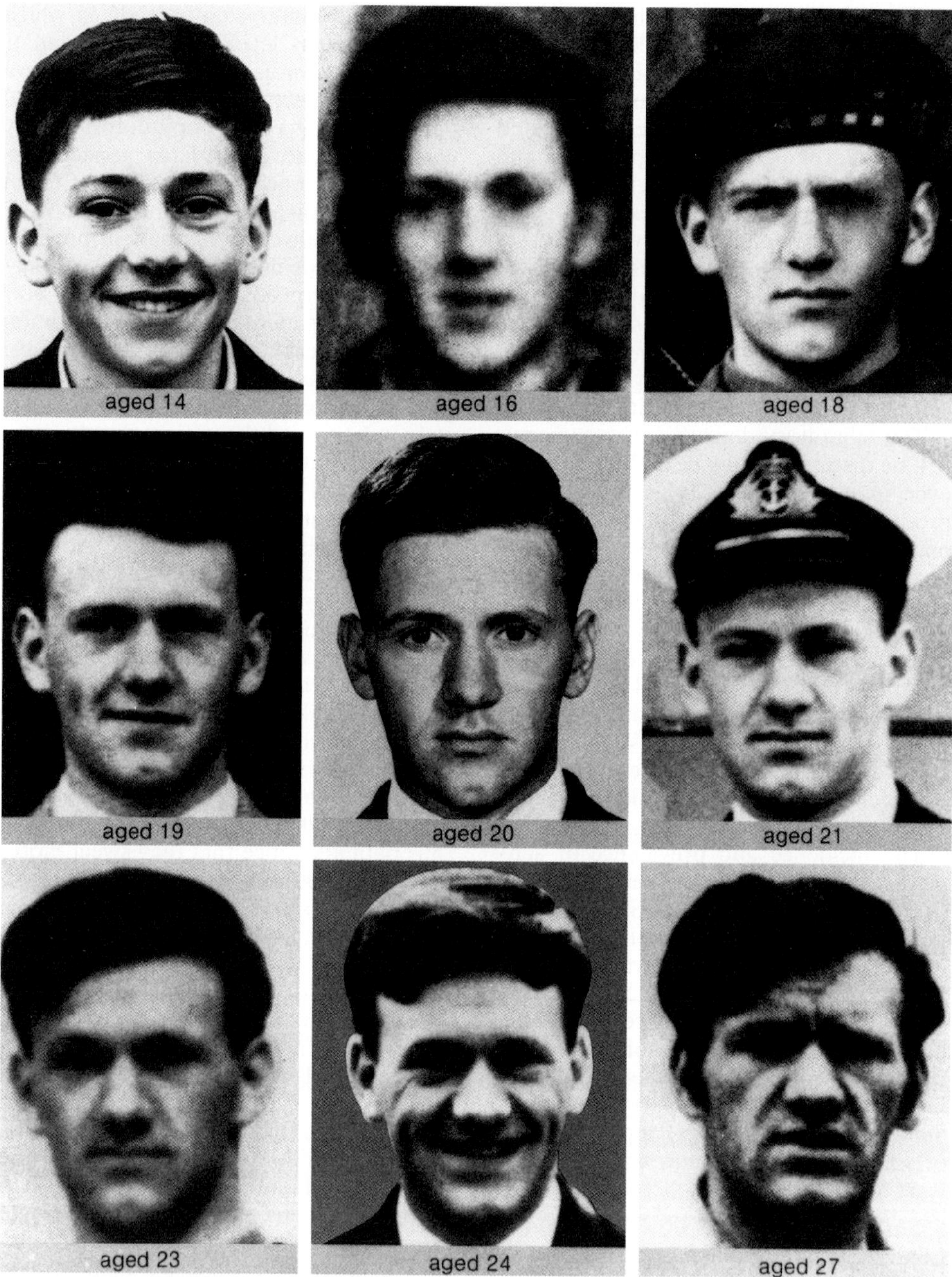

Fig. 2. The change in facial appearance of a patient with acromegaly taken over a thirteen-year period. The development of an acromegalic appearance is seen, with enlargement of the supraorbital ridges and nose, thickening of the lips and generalized coarsening of the features. (Reproduced by permission from [23])

Table 1. Clinical and laboratory findings in 57 patients with acromegaly[a]

Finding	Present/Total
Recent acral growth	57/57
Arthralgias	41/57
Excessive sweating	52/57
Weakness	50/57
Malocclusion	39/57
New skin tags	33/57
Hypertension (blood pressure >150/95)	21/57
Carpal tunnel syndrome	25/57
Fasting blood sugar >110 mg/dl	17/57
Abnormal glucose tolerance test (>6.1 mmol/l)	39/57
Heel-pad thickness >22 mm	48/53
Prolactin >25 ng/ml	8/51
Serum phosphorus >4.5 mg/dl (>1.5 mmol/l)	26/54
Sella volume >1300 mm^2	55/57
Thyroxine <4.1 µg/dl (<53 nmol/l)[b]	0/57
Testosterone (males) <300 ng/ml)	7/30
8 am cortisol <8.0 µg/dl (<0.2 µmol/l)	2/57

[a] Reprinted by permission from [4]
[b] 11 patients were receiving thyroxine replacement at the time of study

The signs of acromegaly include the typical facial appearance with soft tissue thickening, greasiness of the skin, coarse features, increased breadth of the nose, thickening of the lips, macroglossia, and prognathism. In women, mild hirsutism may also occur. Examination of the hands shows them to be spade-like hands with sausage-like fingers. There may be thenar wasting, weakness of abduction of the thumb and loss of pinprick sensation in the distribution of the median nerve, particularly on the palmar surface as a result of carpal tunnel syndrome. Examination of the chest and abdomen may reveal organomegaly. The thyroid gland may also be enlarged either symmetrically or with nodules. The skin-fold thickness is often increased, and the skin, particularly the palms of the hands and soles of the feet, is often moist from hyperhidrosis. Multiple skin tags are frequently present. The testes may also be increased in size in male acromegalic patients. The condition of the lower extremities is usually relatively normal with the exception of signs of arthritis, particularly in the knees, and restricted movement of the hip from osteoarthrosis. The feet are often enlarged, with increased soft tissue thickening and an increase in the heel-pad thickness. The relative frequencies of these clinical findings are demonstrated in Table 1.

Complications — Short- and Long-Term

The metabolic complications of acromegaly, including chemical or clinical diabetes mellitus, hypertension, increased hydroxyproline excretion, and increased collagen turnover, are all a result of the high levels of growth hormone. When GH secretion is restored to normal by removal of the pituitary tumor or ectopic GHRH-secreting tumor, or by medical means, these metabolic parameters return to normal. However, there are a number of long-term complications which occur as a result of the excessive growth of the bones. Thus while osteoarthrosis is often ameliorated by treatment, the joints are not restored to normal. In addition, the compressive symptoms on the optic chiasm are often improved when this is decompressed by removal of the pituitary adenoma or reduction in tumor size during medical therapy. However, if there has been long-term compression of the optic chiasm, then full restoration of vision may not be possible.

The precise nature of the heart disease associated with acromegaly is not entirely clear. In patients with long-standing untreated acromegaly, congestive heart failure is a common cause of death. However, since these patients often have hypertension and/or diabetes it is difficult to determine whether the cardiac disease is secondary to these associated diseases or to a specific effect of growth hormone. No specific pathological findings have been demonstrated at autopsy [10]. However, as summarized by Reichlin [13], cardiac enlargement can be found by echocardiography in virtually all acromegalics, whether or not they are hypertensive or have ischemic heart disease. Impaired left ventricular function is present in some but not all cases. The severity of these abnormalities does not consistently correlate with GH levels and they may persist after restoration of normal GH secretion.

One recent study prospectively identified an increased incidence of colonic polyps in acromegalic patients (9 of 17 had polyps) raising the concern that these patients may be at increased risk for development of colon cancer. A retrospective review of 44 patients with acromegaly by the same authors identified four cases of colon cancer [8]. Two other recent studies have shown an increased incidence of gastrointestinal malignancies in acromegalics. Three of twelve patients had colon cancer in one series [7] and of 48 acromegalics in a second series, two had gastric cancer and three had colon cancer [11]. However, the largest survey of mortality in acromegaly (194 patients) did not find an excess mortality from malignant neoplasms [27].

Prognosis

At least one study has shown that the morbidity and mortality of acromegalic patients is worse than for the general population. The twofold increase in mortality rates was associated with hypertension and clinical but not with chemical diabetes. In male patients, there was an increased number of deaths due to cardiovascular and respiratory disease, while cerebrovascular and respiratory deaths were more common in female patients [27]. Unfortunately there are no studies to demonstrate that treatment of the condition leads to a reduction in this increased morbidity and mortality although, a priori, one would predict that reversal of the adverse metabolic effects of excessive GH secretion would be likely to prevent progression of the disease and, in fact, lead to regression. This regression is manifested by reduced soft tissue swelling, diminished sweating, and restoration of normal glucose tolerance. These changes might be expected to indicate a return to a normal prognosis in terms of morbidity and mortality. The advent of increased awareness of the symptoms and signs of acromegaly, the ease of diagnosis, the increased precision of determining the correct etiology, the advent of modern transsphenoidal neurosurgical techniques (which demonstrate that the smaller the tumor at the time of operation

the better the prognosis) and the use of radiotherapy, dopamine agonist therapy, and now somatostatin analog therapy all bode well for an improvement in the quality of life of acromegalic patients as well as in their life expectancy.

Acknowledgment: We thank Suzan Pezzoli and Karen Dorsey for invaluable help in the preparation of this manuscript.

References

1. Alexander L, Appleton D, Hall R, Ross WM, Wilkinson R (1980) Epidemiology of acromegaly in the Newcastle region. Clin Endocrinol 12:7−79
2. Asa SL, Scheithauer BW, Bilbao JM, Horvath E, Ryan N, Kovacs K, Randall RV, Laws ER, Singer W, Linfoot JA, Thorner MO, Vale W (1984) A clinicopathological study of six patients with hypothalamic gangliocytomas producing growth hormone-releasing factor. J Clin Endocrinol Metab 58:796−803
3. Christy NP, Warren MP (1979) In: DeGroot LJ (ed) Disease syndromes of the hypothalamus and anterior pituitary. Endocrinology 1:215−252
4. Clemmons DR, Van Wyk JJ, Ridgway EC, Kliman B, Kjellberg RN, Underwood LE (1979) Evaluation of acromegaly by radioimmunoassay of somatomedin-C. N Engl J Med 301:1138−1142
5. Guillemin R, Brazeau P, Bohlen P, Esch F, Ling N, Wehrenberg WB (1982) Growth hormone-releasing factor from a human pancreatic tumor that caused acromegaly. Science 218:585−587
6. Ho KY, Evans WS, Blizzard RM, Veldhuis JD, Merriam GR, Samojlik E, Furlanetto R, Rogol AD, Kaiser DL, Thorner MO (1987) Effects of sex and age on the 24 hour secretory profile of GH secretion in man: Importance of endogenous estradiol concentrations. J Clin Endocrinol Metab 64:51−58
7. Ituarte EA, Petrini J, Hershman JM (1984) Acromegaly and colon cancer. Ann Intern Med 101:627−628
8. Klein I, Parveen G, Gavaler JS, Van Thiel DH (1982) Colonic polyps in patients with acromegaly. Ann Intern Med 97:27−30
9. Kovacs K, Horvath E (1987) Pathology of pituitary adenomas. In: Molitch ME (ed) Endocrinology and Metabolism Clinics of North America 16:529−551
10. McGuffin WL Jr, Sherman BM, Roth J, Gorden P, Kahn CR, Roberts WC, Frommer PL

(1974) Acromegaly and cardiovascular disorder. Ann Intern Med 81:11–18

11. Pines A, Rozen P, Ron E, Gilat T (1985) Gastrointestinal tumors in acromegalic patients. Am J Gastroenterol 80:266–269

12. Plotsky PM, Vale W (1985) Patterns of growth-hormone-releasing factor and somatostatin secretion into the hypophyseal-portal circulation of the rat. Science 230: 461–463

13. Reichlin S (1974) Regulation of somatotrophic hormone secretion. In: Greep RO, Astwood EB, Knobil E, Sawyer WH, Geiger SR (eds) Endocrinology (Handbook of Physiology Sec 7), American Physiological Society, Washington, DC, pp 405–447

14. Reichlin S (1982) Acromegaly. Medical Grand Rounds 1:9–24

15. Rivier J, Spiess J, Thorner M, Vale W (1982) Characterization of a growth hormone-releasing factor from a human pancreatic islet tumour. Nature 300:276–278

16. Sassolas G, Chayvialle JA, Partensky C, Berger G, Trouillas J, Berger F, Claustrat B, Cohen R, Girod C, Guillemin R (1983) Acromegalie, expression clinique de la production de facteurs de liberation de l'hormone de croissance (GRF) par une tumeur pancreatique. Ann Endocrinol (Paris) 44: 347–354

17. Soliman AT, Hassan AEHI, Aref MK, Hintz RC, Rosenfeld RG, Rogol AD (1986) Serum insulin-like growth factors I and II concentrations and growth hormone and insulin responses to arginine infusion in children with protein-energy malnutrition before and after nutritional rehabilitation. Pediatr Res 20: 1122–1130

18. Tannenbaum GS, Ling N (1984) The interrelationships of growth hormone (GH)-releasing factor and somatostatin in generation of the ultradian rhythm of GH secretion. Endocrinology 115:1952–1957

19. Tannenbaum GS, Martin JB (1976) Evidence for an endogenous ultradian rhythm governing growth hormone secretion in the rat. Endocrinology 98:562–570

20. Thorner MO, Frohman LA, Leong DA, Thominet J, Downs T, Hellmann P, Chitwood J, Vaughan JM, Valc W in collaboration with: Besser GM, Lytras N, Edwards CW, Schaaf M, Gelato M, Krieger DT, Marcovitz S, Ituarte E, Boyd AE, Malarkey WB, Blackard WG, Prioleau G, Melmed S, Charest NJ (1984) Extra-hypothalamic growth-hormone-releasing factor (GRF) secretion is a rare cause of acromegaly: Plasma GRF levels in 177 acromegalic patients. J Clin Endocrinol Metab 59:846–849

21. Thorner MO, Perryman RL, Cronin MJ, Rogol AD, Draznin M, Johanson A, Vale W, Horvath E, Kovacs K (1982) Somatotroph hyperplasia: Successful treatment of acromegaly by removal of a pancreatic islet tumor secreting a growth hormone releasing factor. J Clin Invest 70:965–977

22. Vance ML, Kaiser DL, Evans WS, Furlanetto R, Vale W, Rivier J, Thorner MO (1985) Pulsatile growth hormone secretion in normal man during a continuous 24-hour infusion of human growth hormone releasing factor (1–40). Evidence for intermittent somatostatin secretion. J Clin Invest 75: 1584–1590

23. Wass JAH (1987) Acromegaly. In: Besser GM, Dudworth AG (eds) Clinical Endocrinology, An Illustrated Text 3.1–3.12. Gower Medical Publishing, London

24. Wehrenberg WB, Brazeau P, Luben R, Bohlen P, Guillemin R (1982) Inhibition of the pulsatile secretion of growth hormone by monoclonal antibodies to the hypothalamic growth hormone releasing factor (GRF). Endocrinology 111:21–47

25. Wehrenberg WB, Ling N, Bohlen P, Esch F, Brazeau P, Guillemin R (1982) Physiological roles of somatocrinin and somatostatin in the regulation of growth hormone secretion. Biochem Biophys Res Commun 109:562

26. Williams T, Berelowitz M, Joffe SN, Thorner MO, Rivier J, Vale W, Frohman LA (1984) Impaired growth hormone responses to growth hormone releasing factor in obesity: A pituitary defect reversible with weight reduction. N Engl J Med 311:1403–1407

27. Wright AD, Hill DM, Lowy C, Fraser TR (1970) Mortality in Acromegaly. Q J Med 39:1–16

2. Correlation Between Preoperative Testing and Tumour Morphology in Acromegaly

D. Killinger, J. Gonzalez, E. Horvath, K. Kovacs, H. Smyth

Departments of Medicine, Pathology and Neurosurgery, the University of Toronto, Toronto, Ontario, Canada

The diagnosis of acromegaly is usually made on the basis of clinical features and an elevated basal growth hormone (GH) level. Most cases have an abnormal pituitary fossa on skull x-ray. In situations in which basal GH levels are normal, or marginally elevated, a failure to suppress plasma GH below 2 µg/l during an oral glucose tolerance test is used to confirm the diagnosis. During the investigation of acromegalic patients, it has been found that hyperprolactinaemia is present in between 20 to 60% of patients [3, 13], and that the dynamics of growth hormone release may be abnormal. A lack of suppression or a paradoxical rise in GH secretion following glucose ingestion occurs in roughly 90% of patients [12]. A rise in GH following stimulation with thyrotropin releasing hormone (TRH) is found in 50 to 60% of cases [4, 16] and an increase in GH in response to luteinizing hormone releasing hormone (LHRH) stimulation is found in 20 to 30% of cases [2, 15].

The high correlation between the increase of GH following TRH and the suppression of GH by a dopaminergic drug such as bromocriptine [7] suggests that the TRH test may be helpful in predicting the response to therapy. The value of provocative tests in the diagnosis of patients with acromegaly is, however, questionable.

In the present study, a comparison was made of the results of preoperative evaluation of the GH response to an oral glucose tolerance test, TRH and LHRH stimulation, and insulin-induced hypoglycaemia and measurement of basal serum prolactin (PRL) levels with the results of pituitary histology. The purpose of the study was to determine if preoperative investigation could predict the histological outcome in patients with acromegaly and also to determine if the histology of the GH-secreting adenoma influenced the surgical outcome.

Patients

Fifty patients with proven acromegaly had adequate pre- and postoperative evaluation. The preoperative studies consisted of at least 6 growth hormone levels taken fasting between 8 and 9 a.m. on different occasions along with the GH response to oral glucose loading, stimulation with TRH, LHRH and insulin-induced hypoglycaemia. Glucose tolerance tests were not carried out in patients with pre-existing diabetes mellitus, and insulin hypoglycaemia was not attempted in patients on insulin therapy. Postoperative studies consisted of assessment of basal fasting growth hormone along with at least three provocative tests. These studies were carried out one month after surgery and at annual intervals during follow-up.

Radiological studies included skull films and, in some of the earlier cases, tomography of the sella and air encephalography. The remaining cases were studied by computed axial tomography.

The GH response to a 75 g oral glucose load was studied at $-30, 0, 30, 60, 120, 180,$ and 240 min after glucose ingestion. The GH, TSH and PRL response to 200 µg of TRH was studied at $-30, 0, 20, 40, 60,$ and 90 min and the GH, LH and FSH response to 100 µg of LHRH was studied at $-30, 0,$ 30, 60, 90, and 120 min. Hypoglycaemia was induced by 0.2 U/kg of regular insulin given intravenously with glucose, cortisol and GH determinations at $-30, 0, 30, 60,$ 90, and 120 min. Adequate hypoglycaemia required a fall in blood glucose of at least

50% from baseline levels or a fall to less than 2.5 mmol/l.

Pathology

All tumours were studied histologically, by immunocytochemistry and electron microscopy. In selected cases, tumours were also studied by immunoelectron-microscopy (Protein A gold technique).

Results

The pathological findings on examination of the pituitary tissue in these 50 patients reveal 6 tumour types. 1) Tumours consisting of densely granulated GH cells contained medium sized, well-differentiated cells with uniform nuclei and well-defined rough endoplasmic reticulum (RER) and Golgi. There are abundant, large, electron-dense secretory granules (350 to 600 nm). 2) The sparsely granulated GH cell adenomas contain cells of variable size and irregular shape. There is abundant cytoplasm with scattered RER, a prominent Golgi apparatus and a conspicuous juxtanuclear spherical body consisting of microfilaments (fibrous body). The sparse secretory granules measure less than 250 nm. 3) The mixed GH and PRL cell adenomas are bimorphous, consisting most commonly of densely granulated GH cells and sparsely granulated PRL cells. 4) The mammosomatotroph cell adenomas consist of well-differentiated tumours with fine structural features similar to densely granulated GH cell adenomas. The size of the secretory granules may be up to 2000 nm. The distinguishing marker is the presence of granule extrusions which in the human gland appear to signify PRL production. 5) The acidophil stem cell adenoma is monomorphous, sparsely granulated and often markedly oncocytic. The cells may show morphologic differentiation toward PRL cells (granule extrusion) as well as toward GH cells (fibrous bodies). Unique, giant mitochondria are frequently seen. 6) Plurihormonal tumours associated with acromegaly most frequently consist of densely granulated GH cells and one or more morphologic cell

types (PRL cells, glycoprotein hormone producing cells).

The relative frequency of adenomas among the cell types is shown in Table 1. Pure GH-secreting adenomas accounted for 44% of the tumours and sparsely and densely granulated adenomas were encountered with equal frequency. Mixed tumours containing both GH and PRL secreting cells accounted for 28% of the adenomas while mammosomatotroph cell adenomas with both GH and PRL secreted by a single well-differentiated cell accounted for 12% of the tumours. There were seven (14%) plurihormonal tumours with cells staining for combinations of peptides including GH and TSH, GH and α subunit and GH and FSH. One tumour was an acidophil stem cell adenoma.

Table 1. The relative frequenccy of the type of GH secretory adenomas in patients presenting with acromegaly

— Sparsely granulated GH cell adenoma	n = 11	22%
— Densely granulated GH cell adenoma	n = 11	22%
— Mixed GH and PRL cell adenoma	n = 14	28%
— Mammosomatotroph cell adenoma	n = 6	12%
— Plurihormonal cell adenoma	n = 7	14%
— Acidophil stem cell adenoma	n = 1	2%
	Total 50	

The mean age of patients presenting with each of the tumour types is shown in Table 2. The age at the time of diagnosis was similar in each type of adenoma with the exception of those containing sparsely granulated GH cells. These patients tended to be younger, in keeping with the reported aggressive nature of sparsely granulated GH cell adenomas [10].

The sex ratio of patients presenting with each tumour type is also outlined in Table 2. There were 30 male and 20 female patients in this study. There was a tendency for an increased number of male patients to have mixed GH and PRL cell adenomas while the male : female distribution of patients

Table 2. Age and sex ratio of acromegalic patients with different types of adenoma

	Age	Sex Male	Female
– Sparsely granulated GH cell adenoma	36.8± 9.9	6	5
– Densely granulated GH cell adenoma	44.2±13.1	6	5
– Mixed GH and PRL cell adenoma	41.3±14.2	9	5
– Mammosomatotroph cell adenoma	41.8±13.1	4	2
– Plurihormonal cell adenoma	44.1±11.0	4	3
– Acidophil stem cell adenoma	53.0	1	
Total		30	20

with the remaining tumour types was almost equal.

Table 3 shows the mean GH and PRL levels in patients presenting with each type of adenoma. The highest levels of both GH and PRL were found in patients with mixed GH and PRL cell tumours, and 8 out of 14 of these patients had elevated PRL levels. The next highest mean GH levels were found in patients with sparsely granulated GH cell adenomas and 5 of these 11 patients also had elevated PRL levels: the increase in PRL was, however, modest with a mean value of 30 µg/l. Hyperprolactinaemia was found in patients with each tumour type with the exception of the single patient with the acidophil stem cell adenoma.

The GH response to oral glucose loading is shown in Table 4. None of the patients responded normally to the ingestion of glucose by having a fall in GH to less than 2 µg/l, and 3 patients had an incomplete suppression of GH. There was a paradoxical rise in GH (greater than 50% increase) in 32% of patients and no change in GH in 61%. The GH response to oral glucose loading did not differ with the type of tumour present.

Table 3. Mean preoperative GH and PRL levels and number of acromegalic patients with hyperprolactinaemia in the different types of adenomas

		GH µg/l	PRL µg/l	High PRL n (%)
– Sparsely granulated GH cell adenoma	n = 11	43	30	5 (45)
– Densely granulated GH cell adenoma	n = 11	40	14	1 (9)
– Mixed GH and PRL cell adenoma	n = 14	62	141	8 (57)
– Mammosomatotroph cell adenoma	n = 6	30	41	2 (33)
– Plurihormonal cell adenoma	n = 7	18	33	2 (28)
– Acidophil stem cell adenoma	n = 1	17	20	– –
Total		50		18 (36)

Table 4. The GH response to oral glucose tolerance test in acromegalic patients with different types of adenoma

		A	B	C	D
– Sparsely granulated GH cell adenoma	n = 11	–	1	2	8
– Densely granulated GH cell adenoma	n = 11	–	1	5	5
– Mixed GH and PRL cell adenoma	n = 14	–	–	5	9
– Mammosomatotroph cell adenoma	n = 6	–	–	2	4
– Plurihormonal cell adenoma	n = 6	–	1	2	3
– Acidophil stem cell adenoma	n = 1	–	–	–	1
Total	49	0	3	16	30

A: Suppression of GH to less than 2 µg/l
B: Suppression of GH to less than 5 µg/l
C: Paradoxical rise in GH
D: No change in GH

The GH and PRL response to the intravenous injection of TRH is shown in Table 5. A positive GH response consisted in a GH increase of more than 50% above baseline, and a PRL response was considered positive if there was a greater than 100% increase above baseline. There was a positive GH response to TRH in 59% of patients and a positive PRL response in 44%. Only 3 of the 11 (27%) patients with sparsely granulated cell adenomas had a positive GH response to TRH, while in all other tumour types there was a positive response in 50 to 70% of cases. There was a positive PRL response to TRH in only 1 of the 6 patients with mammosomatotroph cell adenomas but there were no differences in the PRL response to TRH in the other tumour types.

The GH response to LHRH was tested in 26 patients and was positive in 6 (23%). Of the patients who responded, 4 had densely granulated adenomas. Insulin tolerance testing was carried out in 44 patients and 25 of these failed to increase their GH by 50% in spite of adequate hypoglycaemia. Ten of the 11 patients with sparsely granulated cell adenomas responded poorly to hypoglycaemia and the remainder of the poor responders were evenly distributed among other tumour types.

To compare the relative size of the tumours with respect to pathological diagnosis, radiological classification using a modification of the criteria of Hardy [5] was carried out. Stage I tumours were less than 10 mm and contained within the sella. Stage II tumours were greater than 10 mm and contained within the sella. Stage III tumours showed localized invasion of the sella, and stage IV tumours caused diffuse destruction of the sella. This comparison is found in Table 6. Of the 21 patients with local or diffuse invasion of the sella, 6 had sparsely granulated and 8 had mixed GH and PRL cell adenomas suggesting that

Table 5. Number of patients with positive response of GH and PRL to TRH test in each type of tumour

		Positive responses	
		GH	PRL
– Sparsely granulated GH cell adenoma	n = 11	3	4
– Densely granulated GH cell adenoma	n = 10	7	6
– Mixed GH and PRL cell adenoma	n = 14	9	4
– Mammosomatotroph cell adenoma	n = 6	3	1
– Plurihormonal cell adenoma	n = 7	5	6
– Acidophil stem cell adenoma	n = 1	1	
Total	49	28	21

Positive response of GH: 59% (greater than 50% increase in GH)
Positive response of PRL: 44% (greater than 100% increase in PRL)

Table 6. Radiological classification of tumours found in patients with acromegaly

		I	II	III	IV	Abnormal visual field
– Sparsely granulated GH cell adenoma	n = 11	1	4	6	–	3
– Densely granulated GH cell adenoma	n = 11	1	7	1	2	1
– Mixed GH and PRL cells adenoma	n = 14	1	5	7	1	5
– Mammosomatotroph cell adenoma	n = 6	–	4	1	1	1
– Plurihormonal cell adenoma	n = 7	2	3	1	1	1
– Acidophil stem cell adenoma	n = 1	–	1	–	–	–

Stage I   n = 5   (10%)
Stage II   n = 24 (48%)
Stage III   n = 16 (32%)
Stage IV   n = 5   (10%)

these tumours tend to be the most rapidly growing. Table 6 also shows the number of patients with each tumour type presenting with visual field defects by testing on a tangent screen. Visual field compression was found most frequently in patients with mixed and sparsely granulated adenomas. These tumour types were also found to have the highest GH levels (Table 3).

Table 7 shows the histological and radiological classifications, and the pre- and postoperative GH and PRL levels in the 18 acromegalic patients with hyperprolactinaemia. Postoperatively, 50% of the elevated GH levels had been returned to normal (under 5 µg/l) and 50% of the elevated PRL levels had been returned to normal. In three patients with normal postoperative GH levels, prolactin levels were still elevated and one patient with a normal postoperative PRL had an elevated GH.

The surgical outcome in patients with different types of adenoma is shown in Table 8. A "successful" outcome is a patient who has

Table 7. Pre- and postoperative GH and PRL in acromegalic patients with hyperprolactinaemia

Histologic type	Tumour stage	Preoperative		Postoperative	
		GH	PRL	GH	PRL
Sparsely	III	13.0	35	2.5	33
Sparsely	II	69.0	60	25.0	20
Sparsely	II	12.5	29	3.5	10
Sparsely*	III	34.0	92	2.5	54
Sparsely	III	65.0	34	12.0	6
Densely	II	36.0	41	2.5	8
Mixed	II	222.0	270	57.0	40
Mixed	III	103.0	55	4.0	8
Mixed	III	130.0	40	16.0	9
Mixed	III	122.0	340	33.0	170
Mixed	II	23.0	42	2.0	3
Mixed	III	54.0	277	5.0	20
Mixed*	IV	11.0	820	3.0	610
Mixed	III	39.0	37	9.0	14
Mammosomatotroph	II	20.0	30	4.0	14
Mammosomatotroph	III	30.0	155	25.0	35
Plurihormonal II	II	27.0	40	5.0	6
Plurihormonal*	IV	19.0	170	1.0	112

* Normal postoperative GH with elevated PRL

Table 8. Surgical response in patients with acromegaly

		Successful[a]	Good[b]	Failure[c]
– Sparsely granulated GH cell adenoma	n = 11	3	2	6
– Densely granulated GH cell adenoma	n = 11	6	2	3
– Mixed GH and PRL cell adenoma	n = 14	3	3	8
– Mammosomatotroph cell adenoma	n = 6	5	–	1
– Plurihormonal cell adenoma	n = 7	4	1	2
– Acidophil stem cell adenoma	n = 1	1	–	–

Successful: 43%
Good: 16%
Failure: 41%

[a] Successful: basal GH under 5 µg/l with normal response to testing
[b] Good: basal GH under 5 µg/l with paradoxical response to testing
[c] Failure: basal GH above 5 µg/l

Table 9. Surgical response in acromegaly

		Successful	Good	Failure
Stage I	n = 5	60%	20%	20%
Stage II	n = 24	50%	17%	33%
Stage III	n = 16	25%	19%	56%
Stage IV	n = 5	40%	–	60%

a postoperative basal growth hormone of less than 5 µg/l and all provocative tests normal. A "good" response is a basal GH under 5 µg/l but one or more of the provocative responses are abnormal (most frequently, an increase in GH with TRH stimulation). A surgical failure is a postoperative basal GH over 5 µg/l. By these criteria, 43% of these patients had a "successful" response, 16% a "good" response and 41% were surgical failures requiring additional therapy. The best response was in the densely granulated GH cell adenoma with 8 out of 11 patients having a successful or good response. These tumours tended to be smaller, had the lowest incidence of hyperprolactinaemia and were most likely to have a GH response to LHRH testing. The poorest responses were in patients with mixed GH and PRL cell adenoma (67% failure) and with sparsely granulated GH cell adenoma (54% failure). These patients had the largest tumours, the highest incidence of visual field compression, the highest GH levels and the highest frequency of hyperprolactinaemia. The probability of a successful outcome was further diminished by the fact that one patient with a mixed tumour and one with a sparsely granulated adenoma had normal GH but elevated PRL levels following surgery.

When the surgical outcome is compared with radiological classification a predictable response is apparent (Table 9). Eighty per cent of stage I tumours had a good or successful outcome while 67% of patients with stage II tumours and 44% of patients with stage III tumours had good or successful outcomes. In this series, 3 of the 5 patients with stage IV tumours were successfully operated on – a surprising result, reflecting the relatively small numbers of patients.

Discussion

This group of patients is characteristic of the acromegalic population with respect to age at the time of diagnosis and sex distribution [6, 11]. Examination of the adenoma tissue, removed at the time of transsphenoidal surgery by immunofluorescence staining, and electron microscopy revealed six types of pituitary adenoma in patients with the clinical and laboratory features of growth hormone excess. Sparsely and densely granulated GH cell adenomas and mixed GH and PRL cell adenomas were found with roughly equal frequency (22 to 28%). Mammosomatotroph and plurihormonal cell adenomas were encountered at about half the frequency of these tumours (12 to 14%) and only one acidophil stem cell adenoma was noted in this series.

Hyperprolactinaemia was found in 36% of patients; similar to the percentage noted by Lamberts et al. [8, 9] and Arafah et al. [1]. The highest incidence of hyperprolactinaemia and the highest prolactin levels were in mixed GH- and PRL-secreting tumours. Elevated prolactin levels were also found in 45% of patients with sparsely granulated adenomas, but the elevation in each case was modest. Patients least likely to have elevated prolactin levels are those harbouring densely granulated GH cell adenomas. It is of interest that 40% of the patients with mixed GH and PRL cell adenomas and 70% of the patients with mammosomatotroph, stem cell and plurihormonal tumours had normal serum prolactin levels in spite of positive staining for prolactin in the tumours. Five patients with sparsely granulated GH cell adenomas that did not stain for prolactin had elevated serum PRL levels. The elevated PRL levels in 2 of these patients were seen in the absence of suprasellar extension.

All but one of the patients in this series had elevated basal GH levels. On oral glucose ingestion, three of these patients suppressed their GH to less than 5 μg/l but not down to 2 μg/l. This supports the suggestion by Schaison et al. [12] that the criteria for cure following surgery must be rigorously applied to include suppression of GH to less than 2 μg/l, since suppression to less than 5 μg can be seen in active acromegalic patients.

Provocative testing with insulin hypoglycaemia, LHRH and TRH with measurement of GH and GH plus PRL did not reveal a specific pattern which could be related to the type of tumour. The GH and PRL response to TRH testing was roughly parallel in 50% of the patients with elevated basal levels of both hormones. This phenomenon was found in patients with mixed GH and PRL cell tumours (5) and sparsely granulated GH cell adenomas (4).

The surgical outcome in these patients was influenced by both the stage of the tumours at the time of surgery and the type of tumour. It is difficult to determine whether the type of tumour is an independent variable, since the mixed and sparsely granulated tumours which had the highest failure rate also tended to be the largest, and densely granulated tumours which had the best prognosis tended to be smaller.

These studies show that preoperative testing with currently used tests to modify GH secretion cannot accurately predict the type of GH-secreting tumour. These tests may, however, be helpful in predicting response to medical therapy and postoperative evaluation. Since the surgical outcome in patients with larger tumours is less favourable, they may help select patients who would benefit from medical therapy to reduce tumour size prior to surgical intervention.

Acknowledgments. This study was supported by a grant from the Whitney Foundation. Pre- and postoperative tests were carried out in the Clinical Investigation Unit of the Wellesley Hospital. The authors would like to express their appreciation to Patricia Leahy and the staff of the Unit for their dedication in the investigation and follow-up of these patients.

References

1. Arafah BM, Brodkey JS, Kaufmann B, Velasco M, Manni A, Pearson OH (1980) Transphenoidal microsurgery in the treatment of acromegaly and gigantism. J Clin Endocrinol Metab 50:578–585
2. Arosio M, Giovanelli MA, Riva E, Nava C, Ambrosi B, Faglia G (1983) Clinical use of pre- and post surgical evaluation of abnormal GH responses in acromegaly. J Neurosurg 59:402–408
3. De Pablo F, Eastman RC, Roth J, Gorden P (1981) Plasma prolactin in acromegaly before and after treatment. J Clin Endocrinol Metab 53:344–352
4. Hanew K, Kokubun M, Sasaki A, Mouri T, Yoshinaga K (1980) The spectrum of pituitary growth hormone responses to pharmacological stimuli in acromegaly. J Clin Endocrinol Metab 51:292–297
5. Hardy J (1979) Transsphenoidal microsurgical treatment of pituitary tumours. In: Lifoot JA (ed) Recent Advances in the Diagnosis and Treatment of Pituitary Tumours. Raven Press, New York, pp 375–388
6. Jadresic A, Banks LM, Child DF, Diamant L, Doyle H, Fraser TR, Joplin GF (1982) The acromegaly syndrome: Relation between clinical features, growth hormone values and radiological characteristics of the pituitary tumours. Q J Med 51:189–204
7. Lamberts SWJ, Klijn JGM, Kwa GH, Birkenhager JC (1979) The dynamics of growth hormone and prolactin secretion in acromegaly patients with "mixed" pituitary tumours. Acta Endocrinol 90:198–210
8. Lamberts SWJ, Liuzzi A, Chiodini PG, Verde S, Klijn JGM, Birkenhager JC (1982) The value of plasma prolactin levels in the prediction of the responsiveness of growth hormone secretion to bromocriptine and TRH in acromegaly. Eur J Clin Invest 12: 151–155
9. Lamberts SWJ, Klijn JGM, van Vroonhoven CCJ, Stefanko SZ, Liuzzi A (1983) The role of prolactin in the inhibitory action of bromocriptine on growth hormone secretion in acromegaly. Acta Endocrinol 103: 446–450
10. Melmed S, Braunstein GD, Horvath E, Ezrin C, Kovacs K (1983) Pathophysiology of acromegaly. Endocr Rev 4:271–289
11. Nabarro JDN (1987) Acromegaly. Clin Endocrinol 26:481–511
12. Schaison G, Couzinet B, Moatti N, Pertuiset B (1983) Critical study of the growth hormone response to dynamic tests and the insulin growth factor assay in acromegaly after surgery. Clin Endocrinol 18:541–549

13. Serri O, Somma M, Comtois R, Rasio E, Beauregard H, Jilwan N, Hardy J (1985) Acromegaly: Biochemical assessment of cure after long term follow-up of transsphenoidal selective adenomectomy. J Clin Endocrinol Metab 61:1185−1189
14. Serri O, Robert F, Comtois R, Jilwan N, Beauregard H, Hardy J, Somma M (1987) Distinctive features of prolactin secretion in acromegalic patients with hyperprolactinemia. Clin Endocrinol 27:429−436
15. Shibasaki T, Hotta M, Masuda A, et al. (1986) Studies on the response of growth hormone (GH) secretion to GH-releasing hormone, Thyrotropin-releasing hormone, Gonadotropin-releasing hormone and somatostatin in acromegaly. J Clin Endocrinol Metab 63:167−173
16. Roelfsema F, van Dulken H, Fröhlich M (1985) Long term results of transsphenoidal pituitary microsurgery in 60 acromegalic patients. Clin Endocrinol 23:555−565

3. Acromegaly: Objectives of Therapy

H.-J. Quabbe

Department of Internal Medicine, Section of Endocrinology, Klinikum Steglitz, Freie Universität, Berlin, FRG

Untreated acromegaly is associated with increased morbidity and reduced life expectancy [1, 19, 33]. Advances in microsurgical and radiation techniques and the development of new forms of medical treatment have now greatly improved the fate of these patients. On the other hand, refined methods of endocrinological evaluation have shown that complete cure is still not achieved in many patients [22]. New insights into the physiology of GH secretion and its regulation have been gained. More sensitive methods for the radioimmunological determination of GH and the GH-dependent somatomedin-C (Sm-C/IGF I) have made it possible to better define the limits between normal and pathological secretion. This review will therefore attempt to discuss the objectives of treatment especially in terms of GH concentrations and dynamics of secretion following surgical and/or irradiation therapy or during medical treatment.

Before the development of microsurgical techniques for selective adenomectomy, surgical and/or irradiation therapy was considered when compression of the optic chiasma or basal hypothalamic structures was present or imminent or when headache became an intractable problem. Success was largely defined in terms of tumor mass removal. The transsphenoidal microsurgical approach now allows selective removal of GH-secreting microadenomas in over 90% of cases by an experienced neurosurgeon, but results in patients with larger tumors are less good [23]. Removal of small adenomas can usually be achieved with complete preservation of pituitary function. Larger tumors have often already impaired other pituitary functions and further sac-

rifices may be necessary if complete tumor removal is to be accomplished.

Irradiation therapy lowers GH concentrations to values below 5 ng/ml in about 50% of the patients after 5 years and in about 70% after 10 years. The slow pace of hormone decrease and a high rate of secondary pituitary failure make irradiation a treatment of second choice in patients with acromegaly [7, 10, 23].

Drug treatment is considered to be useful following insufficient operative removal of a GH-secreting adenoma as well as following radiation therapy (until reduction of GH secretion takes place over the course of several years). In selected cases it may be indicated as a primary form of therapy. Medical treatment of acromegaly first became possible with the description of a paradoxical GH suppressing effect of dopamine agonist drugs [18]. However, only approximately 20% of patients respond to dopamine agonist therapy with GH concentrations below 5 ng/ml [23]. The hypothalamic growth hormone release inhibiting hormone, somatostatin, has been shown to inhibit the secretion of GH not only in normal subjects but also in patients with acromegaly [34]. Long-acting somatostatin analogs with increased specificity for the suppression of GH − as opposed to that of other hormones, especially insulin − have subsequently been developed and one of them is now being used in patients with acromegaly [2, 17].

In neurosurgical terms the objectives of treatment in acromegaly are removal of the GH-secreting adenoma with preservation of normal pituitary tissue on the one hand, and decompression of the optic nerves and of other topographically related structures (basal hypothalamus, sinus cavernosus etc.) in cases with larger tumors, on the other hand. In endocrinological terms the objectives of treatment are elimination/reduction of GH excess and preservation/restoration of normal pituitary function. The endocrinological evaluation of treatment success is based on the determination of GH and of IGF I in blood. Hence, a limit has to be defined for admissible GH and/or IGF I concentrations following surgery/irradiation or during medical treatment. On the other hand, the integrity of the normal anterior pituitary hormone secretion is determined by measuring ACTH, LH/FSH, PRL and TSH in the basal state and during function tests.

While it is easy to define the objectives of therapy in general terms, it is more difficult to be precise in important details of GH/IGF I concentration and regulation. This becomes quickly apparent when one reviews criteria used by different authors to define "cure" of acromegaly. Basal GH concentrations below 5 ng/ml, glucose-suppressed values below 2 or 1 ng/ml, reversal of pathological GH responses to TRH, GnRH or during glucose loading, a normal 24-h pattern of GH secretion as well as a normal IGF I value have all been used (for review see [23]). However, none of these criteria − except possibly for 24-h profiles, which are not practicable in routine clinical practice − can be considered absolute proof for complete normalization of GH secretion or the absence of any residual adenoma tissue.

The difficulty to clearly define "normalization" of GH secretion in patients with acromegaly is due to our lack of knowledge of what constitutes "normal" GH secretion in the first place. In addition, the margin between normal secretion and oversecretion that leads to clinically deleterious effects is poorly defined. In healthy subjects, GH is secreted in a pulsatile manner, with a large secretory episode usually occurring early in the night after the onset of sleep [24, 25, 30]. Spontaneous GH peaks can be as high as 50 ng/ml or even higher. On the other hand, during trough periods, the GH concentration is below 1 ng/ml, i.e. below the sensitivity of most GH radioimmunoassays. Until recently, the true basal GH concentration

below that limit was unknown. On the other hand, GH concentrations in patients with proven acromegaly also vary from low to very high values at the time of diagnosis. Most patients have GH concentrations higher than 5 ng/ml, but in some the values are between 2 and 5 ng/ml at all times [5, 21, 22], even when determined by frequent sampling in 24-h profiles.

Because of the pulsatile nature of GH release in healthy subjects "basal" GH concentrations can be misleading in the evaluation of GH secretion in patients suspected of harboring a GH-secreting pituitary adenoma or in the follow-up of patients with acromegaly. A GH value below 1 ng/ml is strong evidence against autonomous GH secretion. However, low GH concentrations between 2 and 10 ng/ml do not rule out the presence of autonomous GH secretion by a pituitary adenoma either at the time of diagnosis or following surgical or radiation therapy. Although "basal" GH concentrations below 5 ng/ml are often used as a criterion for GH normalization following surgical or radiation therapy [23], it is obvious from what has been said that such a definition is imprecise and bound to overestimate the rate of success.

On the other hand, a high GH concentration in a single blood sample may be due to a spontaneous secretory pulse. It is therefore no proof of acromegaly and is entirely compatible with normal, non-autonomous GH secretion (unless the value is excessive, e.g. higher than 100 ng/ml or so). Likewise, a high single GH value does not necessarily indicate the persistence of autonomous GH secretion following operative removal of a GH-secreting adenoma.

In view of these uncertainties in the interpretation of "basal" GH values, the suppressive effect of hyperglycemia on GH secretion is often used as a more stringent criterion. Following oral glucose loading (100 g of glucose, although 75 g have also been used) a GH nadir below 2 ng/ml is usually considered to be sufficient evidence against the presence of acromegaly or for "cure" of acromegaly following treatment [23]. In healthy subjects GH will always be suppressed to concentrations below 1 ng/ml. However, this limit again is arbitrary, being based on the limitations of assay sensitivity rather than on knowledge of the true GH concentration during glucose-induced hyperglycemia. Whether glucose loading always leads to complete GH secretory arrest in normal subjects is unknown. It seems possible that in some patients with acromegaly — especially those with relatively low GH concentrations to begin with — GH may be suppressible below 1 ng/ml, yet not to levels as low as in a healthy person if measured in a supersensitive assay system *(vide infra)*.

In addition to basal and glucose-suppressed GH concentrations, the pathological response of GH to the administration of "foreign" hypothalamic releasing hormones is also used for the follow-up of patients with acromegaly. Approximately 60% and 20% of these patients respond with a substantial GH increase (higher than 50%) to the i.v. application of TRH and GnRH respectively [28, 32]. This is not the case in healthy subjects. Persistence of this pathological response following surgery and/or irradiation or during medical treatment is usually taken to be indicative of persistent autónomous GH secretion [19, 28]. In contrast, a recent report suggests that the GH response to TRH has no prognostic value for normalization of GH secretion or for the risk of recurrence [9]. However, since these authors accepted relatively high GH concentrations as normal (basal GH concentration "below 5 ng/ml") and the follow-up period was relatively short, the matter remains unsettled.

The most comprehensive information on GH secretion is obtained from frequent-sampling 24-h profiles (blood samples usually being taken every 15 to 20 min). Such profiles allow detection of spontaneous secretory episodes, of maxima and minima as well as the calculation of 24-h mean concentrations. In addition they provide information on the temporal pattern of secretion including the sleep-related nocturnal secretory activity. Such profiles have therefore been used to decide whether truly normal GH secretion was present following the surgical treatment of acromegaly and have revealed that this is rarely the case [16].

Calculation of the mean 24-h GH concentration on the basis of frequent-sampling 24-h profiles in healthy subjects has yielded values between 2 and 11 ng/ml, women having higher concentrations than men [23]. Although these values probably represent an overestimation of the true 24-h concentrations due to limitations of assay sensitivity, it is evident that relatively high, mean GH concentrations are compatible with normal GH secretory dynamics and need not indicate the presence of acromegaly. On the other hand, many patients with acromegaly have mean 24-h GH concentrations much lower than these values in healthy subjects. Moreover, patients with insulin-dependent diabetes mellitus have elevated 24-h GH concentrations in relation to the degree of hyperglycemia. Although this may contribute to insulin resistance in such patients, they certainly have no pituitary adenoma and are not acromegalic. Apparently there are large interindividual differences in the mean 24-h GH concentration of non-acromegalic subjects. Individuals seem to have different "thresholds" for the noxious effects of GH excess. Which factors determine whether a given amount of GH in the circulation will cause acromegaly or not is poorly understood. Estrogens are known to promote GH secretion and at the same time inhibit the peripheral action of higher concentrations in women as compared with men. However, other unknown factors must also contribute to the differences in tissue sensitivity to GH in different individuals.

In addition to the total amount of GH available to the tissues, the temporal pattern of secretion is probably also of importance. Although the physiological significance of this pattern — including its link to sleep in man — is as yet largely unknown, there are indications suggesting a role for actions of GH in metabolism and growth promotion. Thus, when hypophysectomized rats are treated with GH, their growth rate is significantly higher when the hormone is administered in a pulsatile fashion as compared with the effect of continuous infusion [3]. The temporal pattern of hormone availability may also be of importance for the action of GH on adipose tissue. In vitro, rat adipose tissue is resistant to the lipolytic action of GH when the hormone is re-administered shortly after a first exposure. The interval during which the tissue is resistant corresponds to the normal temporal spacing of GH pulses in the rat [11]. This suggests that the absence of GH — or at least a very low concentration — for certain periods of time during the 24-h day may be an important factor for a normal effect of GH on bone and in other peripheral tissues. Hence, the continuous presence of even relatively low concentrations of GH may possibly be more deleterious in certain respects than the intermittent presence of relatively high concentrations for short periods of time.

From a diagnostic point of view it is important that healthy subjects always have non-detectable GH concentrations (below 1 ng/ml) at some time during a 24-h profile, while patients with acromegaly do not. Hence, levels of GH concentration below the assay sensitivity — usually 1 ng/ml or a little less — are strong evidence against the presence of acromegaly. Following surgery and/or irradiation, undetectable concentrations in a GH profile are evidence against residual adenoma tissue and against the persistence of acromegaly.

Recently several reports have appeared on the use of more sensitive GH assays for the determination of GH concentrations below the sensitivity of the routine radioimmunoassay methods [6, 12, 29]. Results have shown that GH secretory episodes continue to occur below the 1 ng/ml limit at times hitherto considered to represent periods of secretory arrest. Trough concentrations are apparently 10 to 100 times lower than was previously thought [12, 29]. Hence, all diagnostic criteria for acromegaly based on "basal" GH values, on GH nadirs during oral glucose loading or during 24-h profiles have to be redefined. Accordingly, the values considered to represent "cure" of acromegaly have probably also to be adjusted downwards. However, whether this will have an impact on the indication for treatment — e.g. following incomplete surgery — or for dose-finding studies during drug treatment needs to be further evaluated. Knowledge of truly normalized GH concentrations may, however, allow better prognostic information on the long-term risk of recurrence.

Determination of the plasma concentration of IGF I offers an additional possibility to evaluate the GH secretory status. IGF I is considered to mediate the effects of GH on bone growth. Its half-life in the blood is much longer than that of GH (approximately 3−6 h for IGF I versus approximately 20 min for GH [13, 24]) and IGF I concentrations should therefore mirror integrated concentrations of GH. Circulating IGF I is probably mainly generated in the liver. Recently it has been shown that GH itself has also a direct effect on bone growth and in addition promotes local IGF I generation in epiphyseal chondrocytes [15, 27]. The respective contributions of circulating and locally generated IGF I to bone growth in healthy persons and to acral growth in patients with acromegaly are unknown. It is also not known whether liver and chondrocyte sensitivity to elevated GH concentrations is similar or not. Moreover, other hormones (e.g. prolactin, insulin and steroid hormones [4, 14]) as well as nutritional status have also been shown to influence IGF I generation and/or the secretion of its carrier protein. In normal subjects IGF I concentrations decrease with increasing age [8, 31]. All these influences must be considered in the appraisal of a given IGF I value. Nevertheless, in view of its strong dependence on GH and its longer half-life, IGF I is a valuable indicator of the overall secretory status of GH.

It is generally thought that IGF I concentrations within the normal range are evidence for normalization of GH following surgery/irradiation or during medical treatment [20, 26]. However, our own experience suggests that some patients — usually with relatively low GH concentrations in all tests — can have persistent acromegaly while their IGF I concentrations are within the normal limit. Others have shown that — although IGF I is generally elevated in acromegaly — the correlation between the concentrations of GH and IGF I respectively is poor [20]. There may be a threshold beyond which a further increase of the GH concentration does not cause any further elevation of IGF I generation.

Conclusions

Treatment of acromegaly aims to eliminate the GH excess. At the present time criteria for cure of acromegaly are the presence of spontaneous GH concentrations below 1 ng/ml and/or suppression of GH to concentrations below 1 ng/ml following an oral glucose load. The IGF I concentration should be within normal limits. Although persistence of a pathological GH response to TRH and/or GnRH is usually thought to be evidence of persistent autonomous GH secretion, its clinical importance is controversial. Pituitary function should not deteriorate as a consequence of treatment. Recent GH determinations with supersensitive assays have shown that GH-secretory pulses continue to occur below the sensitivity of previous radioimmunoassays. It is not known, however, whether GH concentrations that are persistently higher than the true basal concentration but below the presently accepted limit of 1 ng/ml are clinically relevant.

References

1. Alexander L, Appleton D, Hall R, Ross WM, Wilkinson R (1980) Epidemiology of Acromegaly in the Newcastle Region. Clin Endocrinol 12:71–79
2. Bauer W, Briner U, Doepfner W, Haller R, Huguenin R, Marbach P, Petcher TJ, Pless J (1982) SMS 201–995: A Very Potent and Selective Octapeptide Analogue of Somatostatin with Prolonged Action. Life Sci 31:1133–1140
3. Clark RG, Jansson J-O, Isaksson O, Robinson ICAF (1985) Intravenous Growth Hormone: Growth Responses to Patterned Infusions in Hypophysectomized Rats. J Endocrinol 104:53–61
4. Clemmons DR, Underwood LE, Ridgway EC, Kliman B, Van Wyk JJ (1981) Hyperprolactinemia is Associated with Increased Immunoreactive Somatomedin C in Hypopituitarism. J Clin Endocrinol Metab 52:731–735
5. Daughaday WH, Starkey RH, Saltman S, Gavin JR III, Mills-Dunlap B, Heath-Monnig E (1987) Characterization of Serum Growth Hormone (GH) and Insulin-Like Growth Factor I in Active Acromegaly with Minimal Elevation of Serum GH. J Clin Endocrinol Metab 65:617–623
6. Drobny EC, Amburn K, Baumann G (1983) Circadian Variation of Basal Plasma Growth Hormone in Man. J Clin Endocrinol Metab 57:524–528
7. Eastman RC, Gorden P, Roth J (1979) Conventional Supervoltage Irradiation is an Effective Treatment for Acromegaly. J Clin Endocrinol Metab 48:931–940
8. Enberg G, Hall K (1984) Immunoreactive IGF-II in Serum of Healthy Subjects and Patients with Growth Hormone Disturbances and Uremia. Acta Endocrinol (Copenh) 107:164–170
9. Eversmann T, Lüdeke U, Fahlbusch R, von Werder K (1986) TRH-stimulierte Wachstumshormonsekretion bei Akromegalie. Therapie-Ergebnisse bei 188 Patienten. Dtsch Med Wochenschr 111:1091–1096
10. Feek CM, McLelland J, Seth J, Toft AD, Irvine WJ, Padfield PL, Edwards CRW (1984) How Effective is External Pituitary Irradiation for Growth Hormone-Secreting Pituitary Tumours? Clin Endocrinol 20:401–408
11. Goodman HM, Coiro V (1981) Induction of Sensitivity to the Insulin-Like Action of Growth Hormone in Normal Rat Adipose Tissue. Endocrinology 108:113–119
12. Hashida S, Nakagawa K, Ishikawa E, Ohtaki S (1985) Basal Level of Human Growth Hormone (hGH) in Normal Serum. Clin Chim Acta 151:185–186
13. Hendricks CM, Eastman RC, Takeda S, Asakawa K, Gorden P (1985) Plasma Clearance of Intravenously Administered Pituitary Human Growth Hormone: Gel Filtration Studies of Heterogenous Components. J Clin Endocrinol Metab 60:864–867
14. Herington AC, Cornell HJ, Kuffer AD (1983) Recent Advances in the Biochemistry and Physiology of the Insulin-Like Growth Factor/Somatomedin Family. Int J Biochem 15:1201–1210
15. Isgaard J, Nilsson A, Lindahl A, Jansson J-O, Isaksson OGP (1986) Effects of Local Administration of GH and IGF-1 on Longitudinal Bone Growth in Rats. Am J Physiol 250:E367–E372
16. Jaquet P, Guibot M, Jaquet C, Grisoli F, Conte Devolx B, Dumas D, Bert J (1980) Circadian Regulation of Growth Hormone Secretion After Treatment in Acromegaly. J Clin Endocrinol Metab 50:322–328
17. Lamberts SWJ, Uitterlinden P, Verschoor L, van Dongen KJ, Del Pozo E (1985) Long-Term Treatment of Acromegaly with the Somatostatin Analogue SMS 201–995. N Engl J Med 313:1576–1578
18. Liuzzi A, Chiodini PG, Botalla L, Cremascoli G, Silvestrini F (1972) Inhibitory Effect of L-Dopa on GH Release in Acromegalic Patients. J Clin Endocrinol Metab 35:941–943
19. Nabarro JDN (1987) Acromegaly. Clin Endocrinol 26:481–512

20. Oppizzi G, Petroncini MM, Dallabonzana D, Cozzi R, Verde G, Chiodini PG, Liuzzi A (1986) Relationship Between Somatomedin-C and Growth Hormone Levels in Acromegaly: Basal and Dynamic Evaluation. J Clin Endocrinol Metab 63:1348–1353

21. Quabbe H-J (1978) Endocrinology of Growth Hormone Producing Tumors. In: Fahlbusch R, von Werder K (eds) Treatment of Pituitary Adenomas, First European Workshop on Treatment of Pituitary Adenomas, Rottach-Egern. Thieme, Stuttgart, pp 47–60

22. Quabbe H-J (1982) Treatment of Acromegaly by Transsphenoidal Operation, 90-Yttrium Implantation and Bromocriptine: Results in 230 Patients. Clin Endocrinol 16:107–119

23. Quabbe H-J (1983) Acromegaly – An Overview. In: Lamberts SWJ, Tilders FJH (eds) Trends in Diagnosis and Treatment of Pituitary Adenomas, Proceedings of the 3rd European Workshop on Pituitary Adenomas, September, Amsterdam

24. Quabbe H-J (1986) Growth Hormone. In: Lightman SL, Everitt BJ (eds) Neuroendocrinology. Blackwell Scientific Publications, Oxford, pp 409–449

25. Quabbe H-J, Schilling E, Helge H (1966) Pattern of Growth Hormone Secretion During a 24-Hour Fast in Normal Adults. J Clin Endocrinol Metab 26:1173–1177

26. Roelfsema F, Frölich M, van Dulken H (1987) Somatomedin-C Levels in Treated and Untreated Patients with Acromegaly. Clin Endocrinol 26:137–144

27. Russell SM, Spencer M (1985) Local Injections of Human or Rat Growth Hormone or of Purified Human Somatomedin-C Stimulate Unilateral Tibial Epiphyseal Growth in Hypophysectomized Rats. Endocrinology 116:2563–2567

28. Schaison G, Couzinet B, Moatti N, Pertuiset B (1983) Critical Study of the Growth Hormone Response to Dynamic Tests and the Insulin Growth Factor Assay in Acromegaly After Microsurgery. Clin Endocrinol 18:541–549

29. Stolar MW, Baumann G (1986) Secretory Patterns of Growth Hormone During Basal Periods in Man. Metabolism 35:883–888

30. Takahashi Y, Kipnis DM, Daughaday WH (1968) Growth Hormone Secretion During Sleep. J Clin Invest 47:2079–2090

31. Vermeulen A (1987) Nyctohemeral Growth Hormone Profiles in Young and Aged Men: Correlation with Somatomedin-C Levels. J Clin Endocrinol Metab 64:884–888

32. Winkelmann W (1977) Plasma Growth Hormone Response to TRH, LHRH and Bromocryptine in Patients with Acromegaly. Akromegalie Studiengruppe der DGE. Acta Endocrinol (Copenh) [Suppl 208] 84:26 (abstract 24)

33. Wright AD, Hill DM, Lowy C, Fraser TR (1970) Mortality in Acromegaly. Q J Med 39:1–16

34. Yen SSC, Siler TM, DeVane GW (1974) Effect of Somatostatin in Patients with Acromegaly. Suppression of Growth Hormone, Prolactin, Insulin and Glucose Levels. N Engl J Med 290:935–938

4. Surgical Treatment of Acromegaly

A. M. Landolt[1], R. Illig[2], J. Zapf[3]

Departments of Neurosurgery[1], Pediatrics[2], and Medicine[3], University of Zurich, Zurich, Switzerland

The results of pituitary surgery, until about 20 years ago, were assessed only in terms of *survival time, working capacity,* and *improvement of vision* [36, 38]. Endocrine improvement could not be documented and, therefore, was not a goal of surgical treatment of hypophyseal tumors. Adenomas situated entirely inside the sella were therefore usually irradiated. However, even in the earliest periods of pituitary surgery, postoperative improvement and, possibly, cure of acromegaly were occasionally observed particularly after transsphenoidal operations. Hochenegg was probably the first surgeon to observe the astonishing reduction in preoperative swelling of the hands and feet in a 31-year-old woman. The change occurred within days of transnasal adenoma extirpation [20, 45]. A similar case was observed by Kocher [24]. This latter patient also noticed that the previous acroparesthesias disappeared within days of the operation. The patient died one month later because of "brain swelling" (?). The autopsy demonstrated an incomplete removal of the tumor. Cushing [5] observed out of 12 patients operated on for acromegaly one patient (case XXVI) who experienced *"not only an immediate relief of subjective discomforts, but the acromegalic manifestations, so far as the thickening and edema of the soft parts were concerned, showed marked amelioration"*. The acromegalic symptoms, unfortunately, recurred one year later. Cushing [5] summarized his experiences as follows: *". . ., it must remain for the time-being a matter of uncertainty as to whether or not, in the absence of a degree of hyperplasia sufficient to cause neighbourhood symptoms, operative measures can hold out any promise to permanently controlling the disorder"*.

The situation changed rapidly after growth hormone (GH) determination by radioimmunoassay became available [49]. New emphasis was placed on surgical treatment of acromegaly by the reintroduction of the transnasal, transsphenoidal approach to the pituitary [14] and the introduction of microsurgical techniques [16]. Conventional sella tomography, fine section computed tomography (CT) with image reconstruction, and magnetic resonance imaging (MRI) allowed the radiologic detection of progressively smaller adenomas.

The primary goal of today's pituitary surgery in acromegalics is the normalization of GH levels with preservation of function of the adjacent normal gland. Transsphenoidal surgery achieves normal postoperative GH levels in 58–90 % of the patients operated on (Table 1). The success rate, however, depends on a number of variables uncontrollable by the surgeon. Tumor size, invasive growth, preoperative GH levels, and previous, unsuccessful treatment are major determinants of the surgical outcome [15, 32, 54]. The preoperative serum GH level determines not only the rate of GH normalization but also the incidence of recurrence [54]. The definition of the upper limit of normal GH levels obviously is of primary importance for evaluation and comparison of treatment result as demonstrated by the data of Quabbe [39] and of Zervas [55] (Table 1). Zervas [55] assigned several patient series treated in different centers to two groups according to the upper limits of normal GH used in the individual institutions. The difference in the cure rates of the two groups is highly significant. No similar comparison of the two groups can be made in the material presented by Quabbe [39] because no center assignment was reported.

Table 1. Acromegaly: Results of transsphenoidal surgery

Author(s)	Year	Number of cases	Number normalized	Percentage normalized	Level of GH used as criterion for normaliza- tion (ng/ml)
Balagura et al. [2]	1981	132	77	58	< 5
Baskin et al. [3]	1982	137	106	77	<10
Delalande et al. [7]	1985	206[b]	98	47[d]	< 5
		126[c]	78	63[d]	< 5
Faglia et al. [11]	1978	18	12	67	<10
Giovanelli et al. [12]	1980	57	47	82	< 5
Grisoli et al. [13]	1985	100	56	56	< 5
Hardy, Somma [17]	1979	120	94	78	< 5
Laws et al. [32]	1982	100	70	70	<10
Lüdecke [33, 34]	1985	222	140	63[e]	< 5
	1987	40	35	87[e]	< 4.4
Quabbe [39][a]	1982	152	83	55	< 5
			121	80	<10
Roelfsema et al. [40]	1985	60	37	62	< 5
Teasdale et al. [46]	1982	28	19	68	<10
Tindall, Barrow [47]	1986	64	45	70	< 5
Tucker et al. [48]	1980	32	24	75	< 5
Williams et al. [50]	1975	59	39	66	< 5
Zervas [55][a]	1987	789	535	68[f]	< 5
		334	299	90[f]	<10
Personal series	1987	169	119	70	< 5

[a] Cooperative studies
[b] Interval 1974−1980
[c] Interval 1981−1984
[d] Difference of the two groups tends towards significance (Fourfold table test, p < 0.011)
[e] Difference of the two groups significant (Fourfold table test, p < 0.01)
[f] Difference of the two groups significant (Fourfold table test, p < 0.0001)

A large number of reports present the short-term results of transsphenoidal acromegaly surgery (Table 1). However, only a few papers describe the long-term results and the incidence of tumor recurrence. Roelfsema et al. [40] controlled 60 patients for up to 7 years (average 3.3 years) and found two patients with tumor recurrence. Additional radiotherapy normalized post-operatively persistent GH hypersecretion in 11 of 17 patients after a mean interval of 2.7 years. Grisoli et al. [13] followed 100 patients up to 6 years. Their cure rate was 78% in enclosed adenomas and 33% in invasive adenomas. No recurrent adenomas were found in patients considered cured at the beginning of the follow-up period. Serri et al. [42] followed 24 patients for 5−11 years. All 8 microadenomas were cured and no recurrences were observed. Normal postoperative GH levels were achieved in 14 macroadenomas. Three relapses were found in this second group. Zervas [54], in a cooperative study, found a recurrence rate of 19 patients in a group of 199 followed for 5 years and 3 in a group of 63 followed for 10 years. Tindall and Barrow [47] rate the prospects of tumor recurrence after an interval of 10 years as very low. We conducted this study to compare our own results in pituitary surgery for acromegaly, particularly in the long range, with the results of the previous studies mentioned, and to evaluate the influence of predetermined factors.

Patients and Methods

A total of 169 patients were operated on between December 1972 and August 1987. A total of 175 surgical procedures were done: 161 patients underwent one transsphenoidal operation, 6 patients had a combined, two-stage procedure involving a transnasal operation and a craniotomy, and 2 patients underwent two separate, transsphenoidal operations done at intervals of 6 months and 2 years respectively because of persistent tumors. Patients undergoing a planned two-stage procedure were counted once, whereas the two patients operated on twice transsphenoidally were counted twice because they were rated as treatment failures. The follow-up period ranged from 1 month to 14 years (average 4.1 years). The last follow-up information from 100 patients (= 60%) was obtained within the last year before evaluation. Eleven patients had died. Fifty-six patients were lost to further follow-up.

All patients were operated on by the same surgeon (AML). The sublabial, transseptal, transsphenoidal approach to the sella, first described by Cushing [6] and modified by Guiot [14] and Hardy [16], was used until 1982 [30]. An endonasal, transseptal exposure of the sphenoid sinus as originally described by Hirsch [19], modified in the light of conservative septal surgery, has been used since [28, 35]. The modified pterional exposure of the chiasm region [1, 18, 52] was used in patients who underwent a combined transsphenoidal and transcranial operation because of tumor extensions that could not be reached by a transsphenoidal operation alone. The transsphenoidal procedure in this situation was always performed first, as suggested by Guiot [15].

Most GH measurements were taken during an oral glucose tolerance test (OGTT). Baseline GH serum levels were used only in a few instances for follow-up studies. Serum GH levels were measured by radioimmunoassay [21]. The upper normal limit in this series is 5 ng/ml. The GH measurement was replaced by measurement of the insulin-like growth factor I (IGF I) for follow-up studies in an increasing number of patients for the following reasons: The patient does not need to be fasting, the values do not depend on stress (puncture of vein), an OGTT is not necessary, and the IGF I value closely reflects the GH value and the OGTT suppressibility [41]. IGF I was determined by

radioimmunoassay according to a previously published method [53]. The normal range is 120–300 ng/ml.

The adenoma diameters shown in Figure 2 were measured either intraoperatively or on preoperative CT scans. Diameters of spheres with identical volume were calculated in the case of adenomas with elipsoid shapes, or in adenomas with irregular outlines, with the help of measurements taken on the CT scans.

Percutaneous high voltage radiotherapy was applied in patients with GH elevations persisting after surgery. A focal dose of 4000 rads applied in daily fractions of 200 rads was used in the large majority of these patients after cerebral radionecrosis had occurred in 5 patients (2 acromegalics) treated with 5000 rads [25].

The new somatostatin octapeptide analog (SMS 201-995, Sandostatin®) was used as pretreatment for 1 week to 2 months before surgery in 13 patients because previously published observations suggested that this may soften the tumor and therefore render surgical removal easier [27, 44]. Subcutaneous injections of 100 µg SMS 201-995 were given at 8-hourly intervals.

Preoperative Findings

The 169 patients were on average 44.2 years of age. There were 96 women (average age: 44.4 years; range: 20–71 years) and 71 men (average age: 43.9 years; range: 16–70 years). The age distribution is shown in Figure 1. Three young men aged 16, 18, and 19 years respectively suffered from gigantism. Their body height was 1.94, 2.05, and 1.91 m. Their abnormal growth had started 2–5 years before the operation. A fourth giant measured 2.03 m, was 24 years old and had a 10-year history of abnormal growth. The 169 adenomas had diameters between 4 and 48 mm; the average was 15.6 mm. The size distribution is shown in Figure 2.

The preoperative GH serum levels were normal (<5 ng/ml) in 6 patients. These 6 patients all suffered from clinically overt acromegaly. The GH values were non-suppressible during the OGTT, and the IGF I values were elevated above 300 ng/ml in all patients. Nine patients had GH values be-

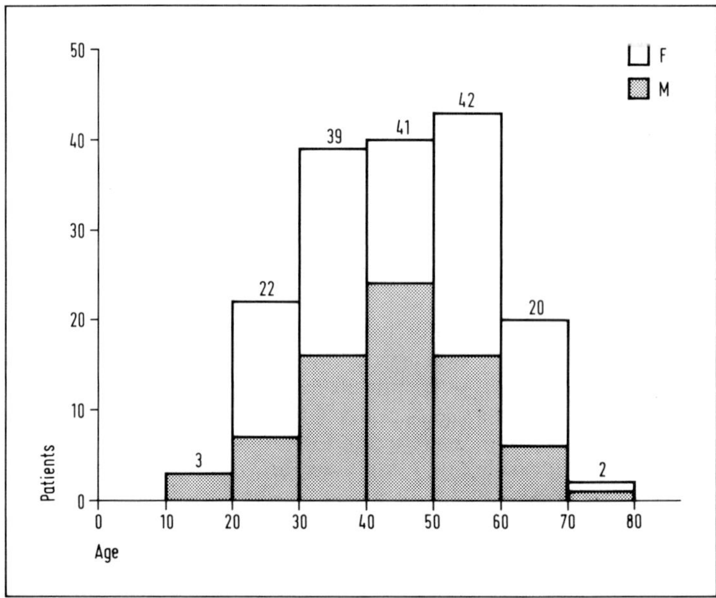

Fig. 1. Sex and age distribution of 169 patients examined

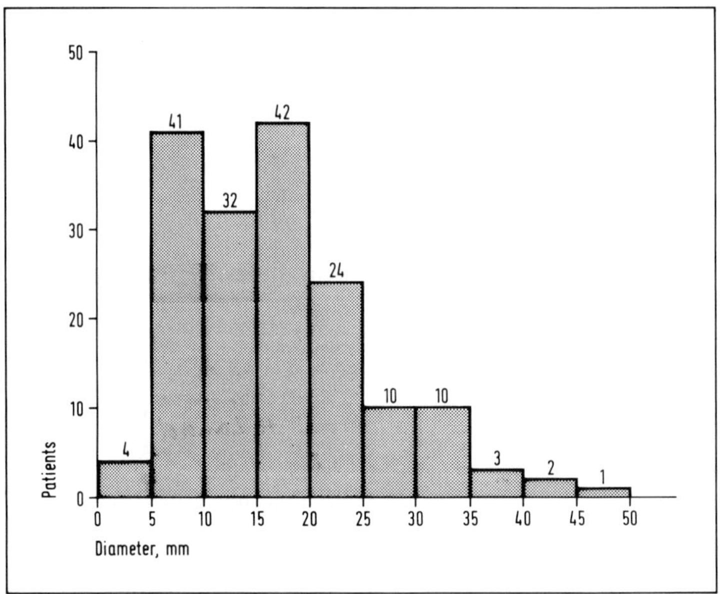

Fig. 2. Distribution of adenoma diameters. Forty-five adenomas (27%) had a diameter of less than 10 mm

tween 5 and 10 ng/ml. The values were non-suppressible during the OGTT and the IGF I values, if obtained, were elevated. Basal GH values between 10 and 40 ng/ml were found in 79 patients (= 47%). The remaining 58 patients had values above 40 ng/ml. The highest value was 336 ng/ml. No preoperative GH values were found in the case histories of 7 patients. Clinically overt diabetes mellitus requiring treatment with diet, oral antidiabetics, insulin, or a combination of these was present in 22 patients (= 13%).

The preoperative GH values were significantly higher in macroadenomas than in microadenomas. No significant difference

Table 2. Acromegaly: Influence of adenoma diameter and invasive growth on preoperative growth hormone level

| | Preoperative growth hormone level | |
	GH < 40 ng/ml	GH ≥ 40 ng/ml
Adenoma diameter ≥10 mm	59 = 55%	48[a]
Adenoma diameter <10 mm	45 = 81%	10[a]
Invasive growth	39 = 60%	26[b]
Non-invasive growth	60 = 69%	27[b]

[a] Difference significant (Fourfold table test, p < 0.0001)
[b] Difference not significant (Fourfold table test, $\chi^2 = 1.3081$)
Note: The sum of the patients is not equal to 169 because the preoperative GH levels and growth type (invasive, non-invasive) were not noted in all cases.

Table 3. Acromegaly: Unsuccessful preoperative treatment

Treatment	Number of Patients
Bromocriptine (Br)	9
Radiotherapy (Rx)	7
Yttrium implantation	1
Surgery	4
Surgery + Br	4
Surgery + Rx	3 (1 personal case)
Surgery + Rx + Br	1
Surgery + Rx + Br + SMS	2 (1 personal case)
Total number of patients	169
Total with previous treatment	31 (18%)
Total with previous surgery	14 (8%)
Total with previous radio-therapy	14 (8%)

was found, however, in the GH values of invasive and non-invasive adenomas (Table 2).

Thirty-one patients (= 18%) had undergone some previous, unsuccessful treatment (Table 3). In the following, only previous surgery and/or radiotherapy will be evaluated. Preoperative bromocriptine treatment, unlike in prolactinomas [26], does not lead to fibrosis in GH-secreting adenomas and, therefore, does not influence the outcome of surgery [8].

Surgical Results

The first postoperative evaluation (within 1 month) of the 169 patients showed normal GH serum levels (<5 ng/ml) in 70% (Table 4). This number correlates well with previously published data (Table 1). The result is somewhat better in microadenomas than in macroadenomas. The difference, however, is not significant (Fourfold table test, $\chi^2 = 1.2506$). Invasive growth of the adenomas, as determined on preoperative CT scans, intraoperative observation by the surgeon, and histological examination of a biopsy specimen of the basal dura obtained routinely since 1977 [30], caused a significant deterioration of the surgical outcome (Table 5). The same is true for adenomas with preoperative serum GH levels ≥40 ng/ml (Table 5). Only 4 of 14 adenomas previously operated on and 2 of 14 previously irradiated adenomas (Table 3) had normal GH levels one month after surgery. Lüdecke [34] has shown that improvement of surgical technique, sophisticated early monitoring of the GH levels, and increasing experience of the surgeon can significantly improve the surgical results (Table 1). Our own data suggest a similar trend. The difference between an early and a late group of interventions, nearly equal in number is, however, not significant (Table 6).

The results of follow-up examinations shown in Table 3 demonstrate that early evaluation of the surgical data is reliable since no deterioration occurs later. The follow-up data reflect a steady improvement of the results. All microadenomas followed up for 4 years or more have reached normal GH serum level. The macroadenomas, including recurrent tumors after surgery and/

Table 4. Acromegaly: Surgical results – follow-up of Zurich series

Postoperative interval	Total number of patients examined	Total	GH $\leq$ 5 ng/ml or IGF I $\leq$ 300 ng/ml (normalized) (number of patients in subgroup)			
			Macro-adenomas	Micro-adenomas	Additional radiotherapy	Additional bromo-criptine
1 month	169	70%	64% (111)	76% (58)	–	–
6 months	134	72%	65% (89)	73% (45)	34% (29)	40% (8)
1 year	126	71%	70% (87)	74% (39)	44% (36)	21% (14)
2 years	108	77%	76% (75)	79% (33)	54% (26)	30% (10)
3 years	86	85%	83% (60)	88% (26)	68% (25)	38% (8)
4 years	77	90%	86% (58)	100% (19)	85% (20)	33% (6)
5 years	64	88%	84% (51)	100% (13)	95% (20)	20% (6)
6 years	48	88%	84% (39)	100% (9)	95% (16)	–
7 years	37	89%	86% (30)	100% (7)	92% (13)	–
8 years	32	88%	85% (26)	100% (6)	92% (12)	–
9 years	27	93%	91% (22)	100% (5)	100% (10)	–
10 years	25	92%	91% (21)	100% (4)	100% (9)	–
11 years	20	95%	94% (16)	100% (4)	100% (8)	–
12 years	15	93%	92% (12)	100% (3)	100% (7)	–

or radiotherapy, achieved a normalization rate of 90% or more 9 years after surgery. This late improvement is caused by the postoperative radiotherapy used in all patients who did not have normal GH or IGF I levels within 6 months of surgery and the few recurrent tumors (see below). This additional radiotherapy reached its full effect after 5 to 9 years, which corresponds roughly to the time course of GH normalization observed after conventional radiotherapy and treatment with heavy particles [10, 22, 23, 31, 43]. The effect of additional bromocriptine therapy was minor and corresponds to the average normalization rate of 24% reported in a survey of the literature [4].

GH hypersecretion recurred in 4 patients after postoperative intervals of 7 months, 1 year, 5 years, and 9 years. All patients had experienced a postoperative period with normal serum GH levels and regression of symptoms. The first patient, a 22-year-old woman, had GH levels of 1 ng/ml 6 months after surgery. The value was still normal (3 ng/ml) one month later; however, there was an abnormal response after TRH. The levels increased steadily under bromocriptine therapy (5 mg/day) and reached 7.7

Table 5. Acromegaly: Factors affecting the outcome of surgery in 169 patients

Parameter	Postoperative serum growth hormone or insulin-like growth factor I level (1 month follow-up)		
	Normalized GH $\leq$ 5 ng/ml IGF I $\leq$ 300 ng/ml	Elevated GH > 5 ng/ml IGF I > 300 ng/ml	Total
Invasive growth	30 = 46%	35	65[a]
Non-invasive growth	73 = 84%	14	87[a]
GH < 40 ng/ml	85 = 81%	20	105[b]
GH $\geq$ 40 ng/ml	30 = 532%	27	57[b]

[a] Difference significant (Fourfold table test, p < 0.0001)
[b] Difference significant (Fourfold table test, p < 0.001)
Note: The sum of the patients is not equal to 169 because the preoperative GH levels and growth type (invasive, non-invasive) were not noted in all cases.

Table 6. Acromegaly: Surgical results in different time periods

Time interval	Postoperative serum growth hormone or insulin-like growth factor I level (1 month follow-up)		
	Normalized GH $\leq$ 5 ng/ml IGF I $\leq$ 300 ng/ml	Elevated GH > 5 ng/ml IGF I > 300 ng/ml	Total
1972–1981	55 = 63%	32	87
1982–1987	59 = 78%	23	82

Difference not significant (Fourfold table test: $\chi^2 = 1.458$)

ng/ml 5 years after surgery. The patient has refused to undergo radiotherapy. The second patient, a 38-year-old man, had a GH level of 2.3 ng/ml without suppression during the OGTT one week after surgery. The baseline level decreased to 1 ng/ml 3 months later. However, GH had risen to 4 ng/ml with minimal reaction during the OGTT one year after surgery. IGF I had risen to 322 ng/ml. The patient, therefore, was irradiated some months ago. The third patient, a 55-year-old woman, had a baseline GH value of 4 ng/ml 1 year after surgery. Four years later clinical signs of recurrence (increased swelling of the face and the hands) appeared. The GH had risen to 19 ng/ml 7 years postoperatively. The patient underwent radiotherapy (4000 rads focal dose). The baseline level was found to be 12.3 ng/ml 6 months after radiotherapy. The fourth patient, a 43-year-old man, had a postoperative GH of 1.7 ng/ml with normal reaction to OGTT 3 years after surgery. The GH level was 3 ng/ml 6 years postoperatively. It remained at the same level of 3 ng/ml 9 years postoperatively. However, OGTT caused a paradoxical GH increase and the IGF I value was 786 ng/ml. One year after radiotherapy and under bromocriptine treatment GH was 2.6 ng/ml without reaction to OGTT and IGF I was 335 ng/ml.

To our surprise, two patients showed spontaneous (?) postoperative improvement of the serum GH levels after an initially unsatisfactory result. The first patient, a 28-year-old woman, had a preoperative GH level of 25.7 ng/ml. The value was lowered to 9 ng/ml by transsphenoidal surgery. Postoperative prolactin was normal. Bromocriptine was used for a period of 6 months and the patient conceived during this treatment. Bromocriptine, therefore, was stopped. The patient was delivered of a normal baby 15 months after the operation.

A control of GH and IGF I levels demonstrated normal values of 2 ng/ml and 80 ng/ml respectively. A last control, 3½ years after surgery, again demonstrated a normal IGF I value of 182 ng/ml. The second patient was a 60-year-old woman. She had a preoperative GH level of 23.3 ng/ml and an IGF I value of 766 ng/ml. She was treated with 3 daily injections of 100 µg SMS 201-995 one week before the operation because she was participating in an experimental study. By error, a post-treatment, preoperative control was not obtained. The first postoperative control, obtained 10 days after the intervention, showed a GH level of 4.3 ng/ml without suppression during OGTT. The IGF I level remained markedly elevated (626 ng/ml). However, the next control, 3 months later, showed a drop in the GH value to 1.3 ng/ml and in the IGF I value to 219 ng/ml. The IGF I value was 287 ng/ml 2 years postoperatively. The possible influence of the pregnancy and of the preoperative SMS treatment in these two particular cases remains unexplained at the present time.

Figure 3 demonstrates the effect of pituitary surgery on acromegaly-associated diabetes. The term "cured" means that no further medical treatment was necessary. A number of patients, however, continued to follow some qualitative dietetic rules for personal reasons. A 24-year-old woman presented a particularly impressive postoperative course. She needed daily injections of 20 U of regular insulin combined with 36 U of long-acting insulin for control of blood glucose. Insulin was stopped immediately after the second intervention in a combined transnasal-transcranial procedure. A diet was no longer necessary and she tolerated even carbonated soft drinks with a particularly high sugar content. Her baseline serum GH level dropped from 8 ng/ml to a baseline value of 1 ng/ml with a normal increase during the second phase of the OGTT. Patients classified as "improved" were able to decrease their dose of insulin or oral antidiabetic drugs.

Thirty-six patients suffered from new or increased endocrine deficits after surgery. Twenty-seven needed substitution with cortisone, 27 with thyroid hormone, 9 with sex steroids, and 2 permanent substitution with

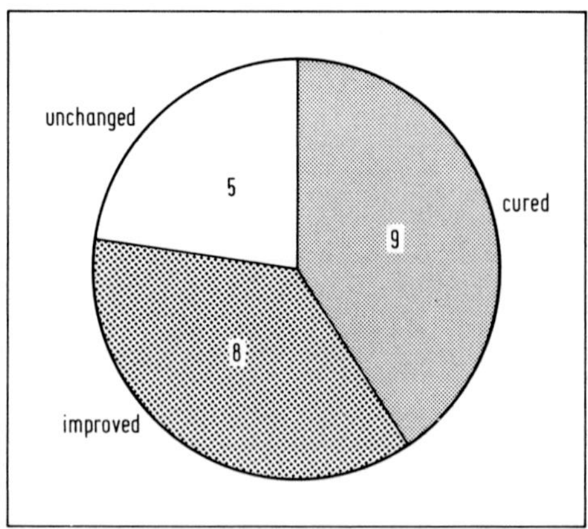

Fig. 3. Postoperative condition of diabetes mellitus. For further explanation see text

vasopressin. Few patients needed sex steroid substitution because of the advanced age of the majority (Fig. 1). One patient, a 48-year-old woman suffering from an invasive supra- and intrasellar adenoma, who had been operated on elsewhere by a transethmoidal approach without evidence of endocrine improvement, suffered from active acromegaly (GH baseline level 10 ng/ml) and from poorly controlled diabetes mellitus even with the combined use of oral antidiabetics and insulin. She experienced a severe visual loss after the second intervention in a combined transnasal-transcranial procedure and suffered from a disturbance of her thirst center and diabetes insipidus, leading to episodes of severe hypernatremia. Her condition improved after successful treatment of the diabetes insipidus with salidiuretics. The GH level was 2 ng/ml, and the diabetes mellitus was cured after the combined procedure.

No other neurologic complications were observed. There were, especially, no further cases of optic nerve damage. Transitory diabetes insipidus, usually lasting a few days, rarely up to 3 months, was not considered a complication because it is frequently present after the use of alcohol as a cauterizing agent in the tumor cavity [37]. Postoperative diabetes insipidus may be mimicked by the well-known phase of postoperative polyuria accompanied by a rapid decrease of soft tissue swelling. The patients may lose up to 9% (average 4.5%) of their preoperative body weight within 3–7 days [30].

Two patients, a 20-year-old woman and a 47-year-old man, suffered from postoperative meningitis. The cerebrospinal fluid (CSF) cell count was 1104 cells/mm^3 and *Staphylococcus aureus* was grown in CSF cultures. The meningitis was accompanied by maxillary sinusitis. The CSF cell count was 170/mm^3 and CSF cultures were negative in the second patient. Both patients responded well to antibiotic treatment. One 45-year-old man suffered four years after transnasal surgery and postoperative radiotherapy from rhinoliquorrhea and recurrent meningitis. All CSF cultures were sterile. The CSF fistula was closed by a second transsphenoidal operation and no further attacks of meningitis were observed.

The postoperative condition of the nose improved considerably because of the reduced soft tissue swelling, and breathing improved as a result of routine correction of septal deviations frequently found in patients suffering from acromegaly. Asymptomatic septal perforations are found in an average of 20% of patients undergoing transnasal pituitary surgery [9]. The incidence of septal perforations decreased to 13% after the introduction of the endonasal approach. Subjective, postoperative worsening of the nasal condition (nasal secretions, nasal bleeding, nasal obstruction, nasal dryness) occurred in 7% of 113 recently re-examined patients [Ch. Gammert, personal communication].

Eleven of the 169 patients are known to have died (Table 7). The death of two patients was related to the surgical intervention. One 49-year-old man suffered from advanced cardiomyopathy. He had severe orthopnea and was bedridden before the operation. The GH level was normalized by the transsphenoidal operation. Cardiac function, however, did not improve. He died from heart failure 1 week after surgery. Autopsy demonstrated complete removal of the adenoma, cardiomegaly, and a few peripheral pulmonary emboli. A second, 32-year-old man died from meningitis caused by *E. coli* two weeks after the second, transcranial, intervention of a combined transcranial-transsphenoidal procedure performed because of a giant adenoma invading the frontal lobe. The route of infection was probably the lumbar drainage catheter inserted for prevention of CSF rhinorrhea. GH was not normalized in this patient. The two surgery-related deaths occurred 8 and 10 years ago. The other 9 deaths were not related to the surgical intervention (Table 7). The most common cause of death was cardiovascular (6 of 11) as in the study of Wright et al. [51].

Summary and Conclusions

Reports from the literature (Table 1) and our own data show that acromegaly can be treated effectively in the majority of patients by a transsphenoidal operation. Only

Table 7. Acromegaly: Mortality in 169 operated patients

Patient	Age years	Sex	Survival time	Postoperative GH normal	Cause of death
1	49	M	1 week	yes	Cardiomyopathy, heart failure
2	32	M	2 weeks	no	Meningitis after craniotomy
3	45	F	1 month	yes	Cerebral melanoma metastasis
4	69	M	7 months	no	Heart failure
5	38	M	2 years	yes	Endocarditis
6	74	F	3 years	yes	Heart failure
7	68	F	5 years	yes	Unknown
8	71	M	6 years	yes	Pulmonary cancer
9	65	F	8 years	no	Cerebral infarction
10	67	F	8 years	yes	Heart failure
11	49	F	10 years	yes	Uterine leiomyosarcoma

a few patients need a second, transcranial, procedure for removal of remaining tumor parts that cannot be reached by the transnasal operation. The mortality and morbidity of the operation are low. Our own observation suggests that both are lowered effectively as the experience of the surgeon increases. Normalization of the serum GH can be obtained in two thirds of the patients by surgery alone. The results in the remaining patients can be further improved by additional radiotherapy if GH levels have not been normalized or if patients suffer from recurrent GH hypersecretion.

GH hypersecretion recurred in only 4 patients. The interval of recurrence was less than 10 years in all cases. This confirms the statement of Tindall and Barrow [47], after an observation period of 10 years, that there appears to be little prospect of tumor recurrence. The size of the adenoma, presence of invasive growth, and preoperative GH levels are important parameters for controlling the outcome of transsphenoidal pituitary surgery. This implies that every adenoma causing acromegaly must be treated as soon as the diagnosis is made. Unnecessary delay, in spite of the extremely slow growth of these adenomas [29], will cause deterioration of the surgical prognosis.

Adenomas which have already been operated on or irradiated have a dismal prognosis. Immediate postoperative endocrinologic re-evaluation is mandatory for detection of patients who need further treatment — either re-operation for further decrease of the remaining tumor mass [34] or radiotherapy.

We currently use preoperative SMS 201-995 treatment. The drug is administered during preoperative phases lasting 1.5 to 2 months and is given in 3 daily doses of 100 µg because this treatment is reported to soften the tumor tissue. Shorter phases of 1 week or 1 month had been used in a first series of trials [27, 44]. We have seen several adenomas which became semiliquid. A quantitative evaluation of the tumor consistency of treated and untreated adenomas, however, is impossible at the present time. A final assessment requires further studies. It is also not known whether this pretreatment will improve the outcome of transsphenoidal surgery. An improvement of the outcome will be difficult to achieve in view of the results presented.

Acknowledgements: The authors wish to thank Dr. T. Torresani, protein hormone laboratory, Children's Hospital, Zurich, for his help in determining the GH; Mrs. Eva Futo and Mrs. Heide Häsler, Department of Medicine, University Hospital, Zurich, for their help in determining the IGF I; Mrs. Mercedes Trigoso, Department of Neurosurgery, University Hospital, Zurich, for her excellent secretarial help, and Mr. Mitchell Bornstein, Basle, for his help in editing the manuscript.

References

1. Adson AW (1918) Hypophysial tumor through the intradural approach. JAMA 71:721–726
2. Balagura S, Derome P, Guiot G (1981) Acromegaly: Analysis of 132 cases treated surgically. Neurosurgery 8:413–416
3. Baskin DS, Boggan JE, Wilson DB (1982) Transsphenoidal microsurgical removal of growth hormone-secreting pituitary adenomas. J Neurosurg 56:634–641
4. Bateman DE, Tunbridge WMG (1979) Bromocriptine in the treatment of acromegaly. Drugs 17:359–364
5. Cushing H (1912) The pituitary and its disorders. Clinical states produced by disorders of the hypophysis cerebri. Lippincott, Philadelphia London, pp 293–294
6. Cushing H (1914) Surgical experiences with pituitary disorders. JAMA 63:1515–1525
7. Delalande O, Peillon F, Maestro JL, Kujas M, Bression D, Le Bouc Y, Le Gentil P, Racadot J, Visot A, Jedynak CP, Derome PJ (1985) Résultats à moyen et long terme de l'adénomectomie sélective hypophysaire dans l'acromégalie. Eléments de prognostic. Ann Endocrinol (Paris) 46:321–323
8. Derome PJ, Kouadri M, Kujas M, Jedynak CP, Peillon F, Racadot J, Visot A (1984) Surgery of PRL and GH secreting adenomas after long term treatment with bromocriptine. In: Lamberts SWJ, Tilders FJH, van der Veen EA, Assis J (eds) Trends in diagnosis and treatment of pituitary adenomas.

Free University Press, Amsterdam, pp 133–137

9. Dobozi M, Landolt AM (1980) Rhinologic late results of sublabial-transsphenoidal pituitary operations. In: Derome PJ, Jedynak CP, Peillon F (eds) Pituitary adenomas – Biology, physiopathology and treatment (Proceedings of the Second European Workshop on Pituitary Adenomas, Paris). Asclepios, Paris pp 241–244

10. Eastman RC, Gorden P, Roth J (1979) Conventional supervoltage irradiation is an effective treatment for acromegaly. J Clin Endocrinol Metab 48:931–940

11. Faglia G, Paracchi A, Farrari C, Beck-Peccoz P (1978) Evaluation of the results of trans-sphenoidal surgery in acromegaly by assessment of the growth-hormone response to thyrotrophin-releasing hormone. Clin Endocrinol 8:373–380

12. Giovanelli MA, Fahlbusch R, Gaini SM, Faglia G, v Werder K (1980) Surgical treatment of growth hormone-secreting microadenomas. In: Faglia G, Giovanelli MA, MacLeod RM (eds) Pituitary microadenomas (Serono symposia, vol 29) Academic Press, London New York Sydney Toronto San Francisco, pp 427–441

13. Grisoli F, Leclerq T, Jequet P, Guibout M, Winteler J-P, Vincentelli F (1985) Transsphenoidal surgery for acromegaly. – Long-term results in 100 patients. Surg Neurol 23:513–519

14. Guiot G (1958) Adénomes hypophysaires. Masson, Paris, pp 157–180

15. Guiot G (1958) Considerations on the surgical treatment of pituitary adenomas. In: Fahlbusch R, v Werder K (eds) Treatment of pituitary adenomas. Thieme, Stuttgart, pp 202–218

16. Hardy J (1969) Transsphenoidal microsurgery of the normal and pathological pituitary. Clin Neurosurg 16:185–216

17. Hardy J, Somma M (1979) Acromegaly: Surgical treatment by transsphenoidal microsurgical removal of the pituitary adenoma. In: Tindall GT, Collins WF (eds) Clinical management of pituitary disorders. Raven Press, New York, pp 209–217

18. Heuer GJ (1931) The surgical approach and the treatment of tumors and other lesions about the optic chiasm. Surg Gynecol Obstet 53:489–518

19. Hirsch O (1911) Über Methoden der operativen Behandlung von Hypophysistumoren auf endonasalem Wege. Arch Laryngol Rhinol 24:129–177

20. Hochenegg J (1908) The operative cure of acromegaly by removal of a hypophysial tumor. Ann Surg 48:781–783

21. Illig R (1972) Wachstumshormonuntersuchungen bei 225 Kindern mit Minderwuchs. Schweiz Med Wochenschr 102:760–765

22. Kjellberg RN, Kliman B (1979) Proton radiosurgery for functioning pituitary adenoma. In: Tindall GT, Collins WF (eds) Clinical management of pituitary disorders. Raven Press, New York, pp 315–334

23. Kliman B, Kjellberg RN, Swisher B, Butler BC (1984) Proton beam therapy of acromegaly: A 20-year experience. In: Black PMcL, Zervas NT, Ridgway EC, Martin JB (eds) Secretory tumors of the pituitary gland (Progress in Endocrine Research and Therapy, vol 1). Raven Press, New York, pp 191–211

24. Kocher T (1909) Ein Fall von Hypophysis-Tumor mit operativer Heilung. Dtsch Z Chir 100:13–37

25. Landolt AM (1980) Hazards of radiotherapy in patients with pituitary adenomas. In: Derome PJ, Jedynak CP, Peillon F (eds) Pituitary adenomas – Biology, physiopathology and treatment (Proceedings of the Second European Workshop on Pituitary Adenomas, Paris). Asclepios, Paris, pp 227–231

26. Landolt AM, Osterwalder V (1984) Perivascular fibrosis in prolactinomas. Is it increased by bromocriptine? J Clin Endocrinol Metab 58:1179–1183

27. Landolt AM, Osterwalder V, Stuckmann G (1987) Preoperative treatment of acromegaly with SMS 201-995; Surgical and pathological observations. In: Lüdecke DK, Tolis G (eds) Growth hormone, growth factors, and acromegaly (Progress in Endocrine Research and Therapy, vol 3). Raven Press, New York, pp 229–244

28. Landolt AM, Schäfer B, Gammert Ch (1985) Die hypophysäre Adenomektomie beim Morbus Cushing und beim Nelson-Syndrom. In: Hauri D, Schmucki O (eds) Erkrankungen von Nebenschilddrüsen und Nebennieren. Fischer, Stuttgart, pp 179–194

29. Landolt AM, Shibata T, Kleihues P, Tuncdogan E (1988) Growth of human pituitary adenomas: facts and speculations. In: Landolt AM, Girard J, Heitz PhU, del Pozo E, Zapf J (eds) Advances in Pituitary Adenoma Research. (Advances in the Biosciences, vol 69). Pergamon Press, Oxford, pp 53–62

30. Landolt, AM, Strebel P (1980) Technique of transsphenoidal operation of pituitary adenomas. In: Krayenbühl H (ed) Advances and technical standards in neurosurgery, vol 7. Springer, Vienna New York, pp 119–177

31. Lawrence JH, Linfoot JA, Born JL, Tobias CA, Chong CY, Okerlund MD, Manougian

E, Garcia JF, Connell GM (1975) Heavy particle irradiation of the pituitary. In: Krayenbühl H, Maspes PE, Sweet WH (eds) Progress in neurological surgery, vol 6. Karger, Basel, pp 272–294

32. Laws ER, Ebersold MJ, Pipgrass DG, Randall RV, Salassa RM (1982) The results of transsphenoidal surgery in specific clinical entities. In: Laws ER, Randall RV, Kern EB, Abboud CF (eds) Management of pituitary adenomas and related lesions with emphasis on transsphenoidal microsurgery. Appleton-Century-Crofts, New York, pp 277–305

33. Lüdecke DK (1985) Recent developments in the treatment of acromegaly. Neurosurg Rev 8:167–173

34. Lüdecke DK (1988) Longterm surgical results in acromegaly. Does the immediate postoperative growth hormone level predict the outcome? In: Landolt AM, Girard J, Heitz PhU, del Pozo E, Zapf J (eds) Advances in pituitary adenoma research (Advances in the Biosciences, vol 69). Pergamon Press, Oxford, pp 243–252

35. Masing H (1980) Management of acute nasal injuries and intranasal surgery. In: Naumann HH (ed) Head and neck surgery, vol 1: Face and facial skull. Thieme, Stuttgart, pp 279–356

36. Mundinger F, Riechert T (1967) Hypophysentumoren und Hypophysektomie. Thieme, Stuttgart, pp 312–313

37. Nicola GC, Tonnarelli GP, Griner AC (1980) Complications of transsphenoidal surgery in pituitary adenomas. In: Derome PJ, Jedynak CP, Peillon F (eds) Pituitary adenomas – Biology, physiopathology and treatment (Proceedings of the Second European Workshop on Pituitary Adenomas, Paris). Asclepios, Paris, pp 237–240

38. Olivecrona H (1967) The surgical treatment of intracranial tumors. In: Olivecrona H, Tönnis W (eds) Handbuch der Neurochirurgie, Band IV: Klinik und Behandlung der raumfordernden intrakraniellen Prozesse, Teil 4. Springer, Berlin Heidelberg New York, pp 254–255

39. Quabbe H-J (1982) Treatment of acromegaly by trans-sphenoidal operation, 90-yttrium implantation and bromocriptine: Results in 230 patients. Clin Endocrinol 16:107–119

40. Roelfsema F, van Dulken H, Fröhlich M (1985) Long-term results of transsphenoidal pituitary microsurgery in 60 acromegalic patients. Clin Endocrinol 23:555–565

41. Schatz H, Starke H, Zapf J (1987) Insulin-like growth factor I/somatomedin C as indicator of activity of acromegaly. In: Lüdecke DK, Tolis G (eds) Growth hormone, growth factors, and acromegaly (Progress in Endocrine Research and Therapy, vol 3). Raven Press, New York, pp 181–188

42. Serri O, Somma M, Comtois R, Rasio E, Beauregard H, Jilwan N, Hardy J (1985) Acromegaly: Biochemical assessment of cure after long-term follow-up of transsphenoidal selective adenomectomy. J Clin Endocrinol Metab 61:1185–1189

43. Sheline GE (1979) Conventional radiation therapy in the treatment of pituitary tumors. In: Tindall GT, Collins WF (eds) Clinical management of pituitary disorders. Raven Press, New York, pp 287–314

44. Spinas GA, Zapf J, Landolt AM, Stuckmann G, Froesch ER (1987) Pre-operative treatment of 5 acromegalics with a somatostatin analogue: endocrine and clinical observations. Acta Endocrinol 114:249–256

45. Stumme (1908) Akromegalie und Hypophyse. Arch Klin Chir 87:437–466

46. Teasdale GM, Hy ID, Beasttall GH, McCruden DC, Thomson JA, Davies DL, Grossart KW, Ratcliffe JG (1982) Cryosurgery or microsurgery in the management of acromegaly. JAMA 247:1289–1291

47. Tindall GT, Barrow DL (1986) Disorders of the pituitary. Mosby, St. Louis Toronto Princeton, pp 217–222

48. Tucker H, Grubb SR, Wigand JP, Waflington CO, Blackard WG, Becker DP (1980) The treatment of acromegaly by transsphenoidal surgery. Arch Intern Med 140: 795–802

49. Utiger RD, Parker ML, Daughaday WH (1962) Studies on human growth hormone. I. A radioimmunoassay for human growth hormone. J Clin Invest 41:254–261

50. Williams RA, Jacobs HS, Kurtz AM, Millar JGB, Oakley NW, Spathis GS, Sulway MJ, Nabarro JDN (1975) The treatment of acromegaly with special reference to transsphenoidal hypophysectomy. Q J Med 44: 79–98

51. Wright AD, Hill DM, Lowy C, Russel Fraser T (1970) Mortality in acromegaly. Q J Med 39:1–16

52. Yasargil MG (1984) Microsurgery, vol 1: Microsurgical anatomy of the basal cisterns and vessels of the brain, diagnostic studies and morphological considerations of the intracranial aneurysms. Thieme, Stuttgart, pp 215–233

53. Zapf J, Walter H, Froesch ER (1981) Radioimmunological determination of insulin-like growth factors I and II in normal subjects and in patients with growth disorders and extrapancreatic tumor hypoglycemia. J Clin Invest 68:1221–1300

54. Zervas NT (1984) Surgical results for pitui-

tary adenomas: results of an international survey. In: Black PMCL, Zervas NT, Ridgway EC, Martin JB (eds) Secretory tumors of the pituitary gland (Progress in Endocrine Research and Therapy, vol 1). Raven Press, New York, pp 377–385

55. Zervas NT (1987) Multicenter surgical results in acromegaly. In: Lüdecke DK, Tolis G (eds) Growth hormone, growth factors, and acromegaly (Progress in Endocrine Research and Therapy, vol 3). Raven Press, New York, pp 253–257

5. External Radiation Therapy of Acromegaly

J. A. H. Wass[1], E. Ciccarelli[1], S. Corsello[1], G. M. Besser[1], N. Plowman[2], A. E. Jones[2]

Departments of Endocrinology[1] and Radiotherapy[2], St Bartholomew's Hospital, London, UK

External pituitary irradiation can be given using either a cobalt source, protons, or a linear accelerator. The intrasellar implantation of ^{90}Y has also been described, but is not widely used.

Prior to growth hormone assays and modern surgical techniques for transsphenoidal adenomectomy, radiotherapy was considered the treatment of choice for acromegaly in many clinics. Exceptions were made in the presence of marked or rapidly progressive visual field deficits. Assessment was based on the evaluation of thyroid, adrenal and gonadal function, as well as on the presence of headaches, visual field deficits and soft tissue changes.

Radiation Dosage

The older data (Table 1) indicated that in terms of control of hyperfunction and visual field deficits, radiotherapy was effective in about 85% of cases, as long as the radiation doses were at least 40 Gy. Lesser doses yielded a lower control rate. There also appeared to be an upper dose limit. Pistenma et al. [8] (Table 1) used doses as high as 76 Gy but found 44 Gy in four and a half weeks was adequate. Kramer [7] increased the dose from 45 to 50 Gy when it became evident that control of GH hypersecretion was slow at the lower dose level but, due to an increase in complications (discussed later), subsequently recommended not exceeding 46 Gy (1.8 Gy per fraction) [3].

Indications and Technique

It is currently advisable to give radiotherapy for incompletely resected tumours and/or for those patients in whom the GH level remains elevated postoperatively. It is also indicated in patients in whom surgery is for any reason contraindicated, being particularly successful when used alone in patients with small tumours and low pretreatment

Table 1. The radiation dose-response in acromegaly

Reference	[9]		[8]	[7]
Calendar time	1942–1959		1956–1972	1957–1971
Number patients	19	18	19	29
Radiation dose (Gy)				
Average	23.3	44	58	–
Range	<35	>35–50	44–76	40–50
Visual field defect				
Pre-irradiation	7	8	6	–
Post-irradiation	4	1	2–4*	–
Hyperfunction				
controlled	5(26%)	14(78%)	17(90%)	25(86%)

* Unclear as to whether 2 or 4 of the 6 patients who had pre-irradiation defects and were treated with irradiation alone had normal fields after radiotherapy

GH levels. Bromocriptine or somatostatin octapeptide should be given while awaiting response to the irradiation.

After construction of an individual head mask to immobilize the patient during therapy, a bicoronal arc rotational technique with wedge filters is used. An alternative recommended method involves three fixed fields (two lateral with wedge filters and one anterosuperior). A modern linear accelerator is always employed. The dose is limited to 45 Gy, as calculated at the 95% isodose line (meaning that no point receives a dose in excess of 47.4 Gy), given at the rate of 1.8 Gy per day. This is consistent with the recommendation of Bloom and Kramer [3]. It is thought that limiting both the individual fraction size and the total dose is important. It should be noted that the optic apparatus of non-acromegalic patients does not appear to have as great a sensitivity to irradiation.

GH Responses to Radiation Therapy

Several studies suggest that the response of GH to irradiation is dependent on the pre-irradiation GH concentration and length of time after treatment. Sheline and Wara [11] (Table 2) found that, if control of acromegaly is defined as achieving a fasting GH level of <20 mU/l (10 ng/ml), patients with pretreatment GH of less than 100 mU/l (50 ng/ml) 17/17 were controlled after 3 years, whereas only five out of seven were con-

trolled when the initial GH level was 100 mU/l (50 ng/ml) or greater. Chang [4] (Table 2) reported a similar experience. Bloom and Kramer [3] found that with a pre-irradiation level less than 80 mU/l (40 ng/ml), nine out of nine patients subsequently had "normalization" of the GH level, whereas this occurred in only five out of eight with initial levels greater than 80 mU/l (40 ng/ml). This also accords with the experience at St Bartholomew's Hospital, where data are available on 27 patients with pretreatment growth hormone values of <50 mU/l and 43 with values above this. In 70.4% of the former group, but in only 37.2% of the latter group, were growth hormone levels of <10 mU/l eventually obtained. In patients with basal growth hormone levels of <50 mU/l, a growth hormone of <10 mU/l occurred in a significantly shorter time than in patients whose growth hormone levels started >50 mU/l (4.8 ± 0.4 years vs 7.05 ± 0.6 years).

We have also studied a sub-group of 31 acromegalic patients, all of whom were regularly followed up for 10 years. A progressive increase in the number of patients reaching serum growth hormone levels of <10 mU/l (20 patients, 64.5%, at 10 years) was observed. In this group the percentage fall in growth hormone was calculated. The maximum effectiveness of radiotherapy in lowering growth hormone levels was observed one year after treatment (53% of pretreatment values). This was followed by a gradual decrease in the rate of fall which persisted after the eighth year of assess-

Table 2. The response to radiation therapy as a function of the initial GH level

Initial GH (mU/l)	Interval (years)	Sheline and Wara [11] (>40 Gy)		Chang [4] (50 Gy)	
		<20	<10	<20	<10
<100	1	8/21	2/21	–	–
	1½	–	–	4/6	1/6
	2	19/23	9/23	–	–
	3	17/17	11/17	–	–
	6	–	–	6/6	5/6
>100	1	5/10	4/10	–	–
	1½	–	–	0/5	0/5
	2	5/ 9	4/ 9	–	–
	3	5/ 7	4/ 7	–	–
	6	–	–	2/3	1/3

ment. A further sub-group of 18 patients followed after treatment for more than 10 years showed a significant reduction in growth hormone levels 11−15 years after radiotherapy. In 3 of these patients growth hormone levels of <10 mU/l were observed for the first time 12−14 years after radiotherapy.

Eastman et al. [5] (Table 3) reported one of the larger series treated primarily with radiotherapy subsequent to availability of the GH assay. Their series contained 47 patients, of whom 16 were followed for 10 years or longer. The mean decrease in plasma GH level was 52% at two years and 77% five years after irradiation. When 20 mU/l (10 ng/ml) was accepted as the upper normal limit, the control increased from 38% at two years to 73% at five years and 81% by 10 years.

Several studies (Table 4) indicate that radiotherapy also is effective in patients

Table 3. The results of megavoltage irradiation (40−50 Gy) when used as sole primary therapy. (Data from [5])

	Initial	2 years	5 years	10 years
No. patients evaluated	47	42	33	16
Decreased plasma GH* mean	−	52%	77%	77%
<20 mU/l	6 (13%)	16 (38%)	24 (73%)	13 (81%)
<10 mU/l	1 (2%)	7 (17%)	14 (42%)	11 (69%)
Hypothyroid	4 (9%)	6 (14%)	4 (12%)	3 (19%)
Hypoadrenal	3 (6%)	5 (12%)	10 (30%)	6 (38%)
Hypogonadal				
Male	4 (13%)	7 (32%)	7 (41%)	7 (58%)
Female	4 (19%)	5 (29%)	7 (44%)	2 (50%)

* Initial range: 10 to 500 mU/l; mean 120 mU/l

Table 4. The results of radiation therapy given for surgical failures

Institution	Surgical technique	Number of patients irradiated	Post-radiotherapy Interval (years)	Post-radiotherapy Remission (GH<20 mU/l)
University of	Cryohypophysectomy	7	2	4
California,	Transfrontal	4	2	3
San Francisco	Transsphenoidal	16	<1 to 10	16
National Institutes of Health	Transfrontal	5	2	4
Middlesex Hospital, London	Transsphenoidal	6	?	4
Karolinska Institute, Stockholm	18 Transsphenoidal 1 Transfrontal	19	1 to 10	16*
Total		57		47 (82%)

* 10 patients reduced to <10 mU/l

References

UCSF:	[2, 10]	Middlesex:	[14]
NIH:	[5]	Karolinska:	[13]

who fail to have their GH levels normalized by a surgical procedure. Pooling data from these studies using 20 mU/l (10 ng/ml) as the normal limit gives a control rate of 82%. Werner et al. [13] who gave radiotherapy four months to ten years after unsuccessful surgery, had an 84% remission rate (53% if 10 mU/l [5 ng/ml] is used as the definition of remission). Interestingly, with isolated GH hypersecretion the one- and ten-year control rates were 42% and 60% respectively, but, if concomitant hyperprolactinaemia was present, the control increased to 70 and 88% at these time intervals. However, this experience has not been found at St Bartholomew's Hospital, where no significant difference was observed in terms of the growth hormone response to radiotherapy between basally normal and hyperprolactinaemic patients. Thus, serum growth hormone levels of <10 mU/l were achieved in 9 out of 27 (33%) of initially normoprolactinaemic and in 15 out of 34 (44%) of initially hyperprolactinaemic patients.

At our institution, external radiotherapy is only given to a patient whose tumour is entirely intrasellar. In none of the 73 patients we have studied and followed for up to 15 years has tumour expansion occurred, and in the majority of patients scanned after radiotherapy a partially empty sella is found.

Unwanted Effects of Radiation Therapy

With modern radiotherapy, in which the high-dose volume is limited to the sella and immediate parasellar region, the main complications of radiation therapy are limited to effects on pituitary function (Table 3) and the optic nerves/chiasm (Table 5). With radiotherapy as the primary treatment, Eastman et al. [5] reported a 10% increase in the incidence of hypothyroidism 10 years after treatment. In the same interval, hypoadrenalism increased from 6 to 38%. There was a similar increase in the rate of hypogonadism. It should be noted that, if laboratory tests were equivocal, or their timing uncertain, Eastman et al. recorded the result as hypofunction, and attributed it to the post-irradiation period. In patients treated (50 Gy at 1.8 Gy per day) at the Karolinska Institute, after failure of an operative procedure to control acromegaly, there was a high incidence of pre-irradiation hypofunction [13]. It ranged from 24% for hypothyroidism to 44% for hypogonadism. After irradiation, the hypofunction rate increased progressively with time. Although panhypopituitarism was "100%" after 10 years, this represented only two patients, hence, the accuracy of the estimate is open to question. The experience at St Bartholomew's Hospital confirms that pituitary replacement therapy is not invariably needed 10 years after treatment. At a mean of 5.7 years after radiotherapy, 25% of patients require replacement therapy [12]. Baskin et al. [2] reported that 71% of patients undergoing transsphenoidal surgery followed by postoperative irradiation developed hypopituitarism, and in 50% this amounted to panhypopituitarism. Feek et al. [6] reported 16, 30, and 47% loss of thyrotrophin, corticotrophin, and gonadotrophin function by 10 years for patients treated with surgery

Table 5. Reported instances of decreased vision after radiation therapy for acromegaly

	Number patients treated	Dose/fraction (Gy)	Impaired vision
Sheline et al. [9]	18	35−50/1.8	1
Eastman et al. [5]	47	40/3.0 to 50/2.0	1
Werner et al. [13]	25	50/1.8	None
Pistenma et al. [8]	19	44−76/2.0	2
Chang [4]	35	50/2.0	1
Aloia et al. [1]	10	55/2.0	None
Bloom and Kramer [3]	40	45−50/1.8−2.2	5
Total	194		10

alone. For patients treated with surgery plus radiotherapy the rates were 38, 54, and 70% respectively. These studies indicate a substantial rate of hypopituitarism following radiotherapy, which is progressive with time and is increased by combining surgery and irradiation.

We and others have assessed prolactin levels after radiotherapy. In our whole group of patients studied 2−5 years after radiotherapy, different patterns in prolactin behaviour were identified. In previously surgically untreated patients, an increase in prolactin levels was observed in 22 out of 23 patients who had normal levels before radiotherapy, and in 17 out of 27 with hyperprolactinaemia initially. In contrast, 10 out of 27 with elevated pre-radiotherapy levels (all >1000 mU/l) had a reduction in prolactin levels. In those patients who had a rise in prolactin levels a progressive fall was seen after a mean of 4 years. No correlation was found between pretreatment prolactin levels and final GH values. No relationship was found between changes in prolactin and the development of hypopituitarism. These data show that different patterns of prolactin behaviour may be identified in acromegalic patients after radiotherapy, suggesting that treatment may produce hyperprolactinaemia from mild hypothalamic damage or conversely may ablate prolactin secreting cells if these were present in the tumour.

In a collected series of 194 patients with acromegaly (Table 5) there were reported instances of impaired vision following irradiation. In three of these [8, 9] impairment was due to tumour progression. The patient of Eastman et al. [5] apparently was treated contrary to general protocol and received 56 Gy at 2 Gy per day. This patient also had systemic sarcoidosis with progressive dementia and retinal lesions characteristic of the uveal form of sarcoidosis, and it was uncertain as to whether the visual impairment resulted from irradiation or sarcoidosis. Chang's patient [4] received 55 Gy at 2.2 Gy per day, again contrary to the general policy at the institution. Three of the five patients of Bloom and Kramer [3] received 50 Gy. Thus there were only two patients with doses of 46 Gy or less who developed visual impairment. Furthermore, in most reports it is unclear as to whether the stated dose is the maximum dose delivered or represents that calculated at some isodose line; with certain older irradiation techniques the actual dose to the optic chiasm significantly exceeds that to the pituitary.

Management of Acromegalics

Most acromegalics have either mixed GH- and PRL-secreting tumours (35%) or pituitary lesions that secrete GH alone. Clinical experience suggests that there is a spectrum of disease ranging from young patients who often have very large tumours associated with very high levels of GH which behave fairly aggressively, to older patients at the other end of the spectrum who have a much smaller tumour and lower levels of GH; these tend to progress more slowly. Earlier debates suggesting that all patients should be treated with only one modality are no longer tenable. Often all three modalities of treatment may be needed in a single patient, particularly the younger ones with aggressive tumours.

It is clear that surgery results in a rapid fall in GH levels but equally it is not always successful, particularly in patients with larger tumours in whom there is a significant incidence of surgically induced hypopituitarism. External pituitary irradiation, although eventually effective in the majority, takes some time to work and bromocriptine, although being extremely effective in some patients, only rarely reduces GH levels to normal. Somatostatin octapeptide is more frequently effective. In the past the treatment advised depended on the local expertise. With more widely available surgery and radiotherapy, this should no longer be the case.

If a patient presents with a large extrasellar tumour, particularly if this is a mixed GH- and PRL-secreting lesion, it is best to try to decrease the size of the tumour first with bromocriptine. This clearly needs extremely careful monitoring of tumour size and visual fields. Surgery should be contemplated at the end of three to six months and is absolutely indicated if there is no change in the size of the tumour, if GH levels remain high or if there is extrasellar extension to the tumour. In these circumstances, surgery may not be curative and radiotherapy has to be advised postoperatively in order to achieve a remission of abnormal GH secretion. In these circumstances, a somatostatin analogue, if effective, or bromocriptine has to be administered in the interim period until the radiotherapy has been fully effective.

In patients with tumours entirely confined to the sella turcica a choice of therapy is available. In competent hands, surgery is most likely to cause a return of GH secretion to normal most rapidly, and radiotherapy is reserved for those patients in whom a surgical cure is not achieved. It is clear that radiotherapy is most rapidly effective in patients with small lesions associated with minimal elevation of GH. Such patients and those who are unwilling to undergo operation may be treated with radiotherapy together with somatostatin octapeptide (Sandostatin®) or bromocriptine, withdrawn at intervals to assess whether the radiotherapy has been fully effective.

Medical treatment of acromegaly alone is rarely indicated except in those patients who are too old or unwilling to undergo ablative therapy to the pituitary.

Conclusion

Acromegaly remains a stubborn therapeutic challenge. The results of surgical management continue to improve with both more widespread acquisition of expertise and advances in techniques and patient selection. Currently though, it is unclear whether prior medical therapy alters the effect of surgery either with regard to its cure rate or its complication rate. Furthermore, the long-term recurrence rate after surgery is not known and, particularly in those with minimal elevation of GH postoperatively, the exact biochemical indications for postoperative irradiation are uncertain. Lastly it is hoped that better medical treatment of the disease will become available and that the present optimism for treatment with long-acting somatostatin analogues will be realized.

References

1. Aloia JF, Roginsky MS, Archambeau JO (1974) Pituitary irradiation in acromegaly. Am J Med Sci 267:81–87
2. Baskin DS, Boggan JE, Wilson CB (1982) Transsphenoidal microsurgical removal of growth hormone secreting pituitary tumours. A review of 137 cases. J Neurosurg 56:634–641
3. Bloom B, Kramer S (1984) Conventional radiation therapy in the management of acromegaly. In: Black P, et al. (eds) Secretory Tumours of the Pituitary Gland (Progress in Endocrine Research and Therapy, vol 1). Raven Press, New York, pp 179–190
4. Chang CH (1982) Radiotherapy of secretory and nonsecretory pituitary adenomas. In: Tumours of the Central Nervous System: Modern Radiotherapy in Multidisciplinary Management. Mason, New York, pp 201–213
5. Eastman RC, Gorden P, Roth J (1979) Conventional supervoltage irradiation is an effective treatment for acromegaly. J Clin Endocrinol Metab 48:931–940
6. Feek CM, McLelland J, Seth J, et al. (1984) How effective is external pituitary irradiation for growth hormone-secreting pituitary tumours? Clin Endocrinol 20:401–408
7. Kramer S (1973) Indications for, and results of, treatment of pituitary tumours by external radiation. In: Kohler PO, Ross GT (eds) Diagnosis and Treatment of Pituitary Tumours. Excerpta Medica/American Elsevier, New York, pp 217–233
8. Pistenma DA, Goffinet DR, Bagshaw MA, Hanbery JW, Eltringham JR (1976) Treatment of acromegaly with megavoltage radiation therapy. Int J Radiat Oncol Biol Phys 1:885–893
9. Sheline GE, Goldberg MB, Feldman R (1961) Pituitary irradiation for acromegaly. Radiology 76:70–75
10. Sheline GE, Tyrell B (1983) Pituitary adenomas. In: Pistenma DA, Phillips TL (eds) Radiation Oncology Annual 1983. Raven Press, New York, pp 1–35
11. Sheline GE, Wara WM (1975) Radiation therapy of acromegaly and nonsecretory chromophobe adenomas of the pituitary. In: Seydel HG (ed) Tumours of the Nervous System. Wiley, New York, pp 117–132
12. Wass JAH, Plowman PN, Jones AE, Besser GM (1987) The treatment of acromegaly by external pituitary irradiation and drugs. In: International Symposium: Challenges of Hypersecretion: Human Growth Hormone. Raven Press, New York, pp 199–206
13. Werner S, Trample EA, Palacios P, Lax I,

Hall K (1985) Growth hormone producing pituitary adenomas with concomitant hypersecretion of prolactin are particularly sensitive to proton irradiation. Int J Radiat Oncol Biol Phys 11:1713−1720

14. Williams RA, Jacobs HS, Kurtz AB, et al. (1975) The treatment of acromegaly with special reference to trans-sphenoidal hypophysectomy. Q J Med 44:79−98

6. Bromocriptine Treatment of Acromegaly

K. von Werder

Medizinische Klinik Innenstadt, Universität München, FRG

Refinement of microsurgical techniques and improvement in applying high radiation dosages selectively to the sella turcica have made transsphenoidal surgery the accepted therapy of choice in acromegaly, followed by high voltage radiotherapy [5, 7, 15, 19]. However, though this has led to considerable improvement of therapeutical results, acromegaly is still a "stubborn therapeutic challenge" as Daughaday pointed out 17 years ago [4]. Thus medical therapy with either dopamine agonists [1] or, more recently, somatostatin analogues [10] have become important alternatives or additional tools in the therapeutic management of active acromegaly [19].

Several drugs have been proposed for the treatment of acromegaly. Estrogens, high doses of progestins, chlorpromazine and other dopamine antagonists have been examined. However, none of these drugs were shown to be effective in lowering GH levels sufficiently. Liuzzi made the observation that L-dopa and dopamine agonists led to a paradoxical reduction of growth hormone levels in more than 50% of acromegalic patients [12]. In normal subjects L-dopa, which is rapidly converted in the hypothalamus into norepinephrine and dopamine, stimulates GHRH release and growth hormone secretion. In acromegalics however, the inhibitory effect on GH release is mediated by direct stimulation of dopamine receptors at the pituitary somatotroph [16]. This is indicated by the fact that after successful pituitary surgery the paradoxical decrease of GH after L-dopa is converted into a regular response with an increase of the GH levels after L-dopa ingestion [7].

Selection of Patients

There is still controversy about the value of GH suppression after acute dopamine agonist administration as a predictor of the response to long-term treatment. Lamberts et al. have shown that patients with acromegaly and elevated prolactin levels have a more pronounced decrease of the GH levels after acute administration of 2.5 mg bromocriptine than those patients with normal prolactin levels [9]. The hyperprolactinaemic patients also show a more pronounced inappropriate GH response to TRH, suggesting that this test may have a predictive value in respect of bromocriptine responsiveness [9].

Since acromegalic patients with an inappropriate rise of GH after TRH are also those patients who show an inappropriate prolactin rise after GHRH [14], i.e. growth hormone behaves prolactin-like and prolactin behaves growth hormone-like, it may be concluded that these patients harbour so-called somatomammotrophic tumours, which are particularly sensitive to bromocriptine [16].

Bromocriptine Dosage

Bromocriptine, which has been shown to be highly effective in the treatment of hyperprolactinaemia, has been widely used for the treatment of acromegaly [1–3, 17, 19–21]. Some authors have proposed the administration of very high dosages up to 90 mg/day [1], though other authors feel that bromocriptine dosages above 20 mg/day do not lead to better results in respect to lowering GH levels [2, 17].

Treatment Results

Besser et al. [1] have reported GH levels below 5 ng/ml in 19% and GH levels below 10 ng/ml in 78% on high-dose bromocriptine therapy. However, the same group reported that 94% of their patients responded clinically with, for example, a decrease in finger circumference during bromocriptine treatment. This discrepancy between biochemical and clinical improvement has also been observed by us and other investigators [2, 7, 19].

We attempted to elucidate the mechanism to explain the discrepancy between biochemical and clinical improvement [6].

We like others [1] have examined the changes in molecular heterogeneity of growth hormone before and after bromocriptine administration. Growth hormone circulates in a monomeric as well as a dimeric form — "big" growth hormone — and a small fraction which elutes with the void volume — "big-big" growth hormone. After bromocriptine administration preferential suppression of the monomeric GH fraction has been observed (Fig. 1).

Since the monomeric fraction is more active in the radioreceptor assay than the dimeric fraction, whereas there is no such difference between the various fractions in respect of their immunological activity, pref-

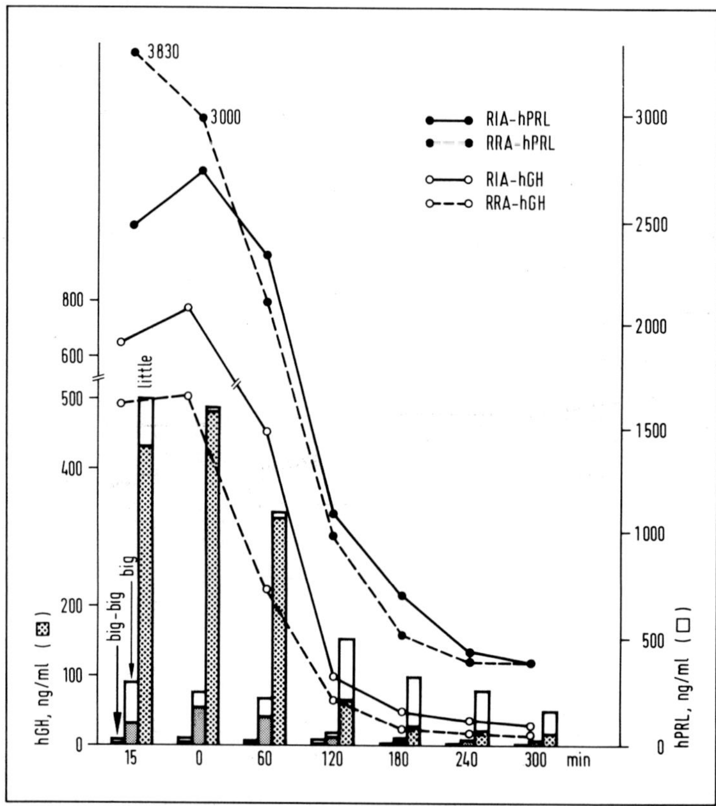

Fig. 1. Growth hormone and prolactin profiles in a 56-year-old patient with a GH- and PRL-producing adenoma after 5 mg bromocriptine p.o. Both hormones were measured by radioimmunoassay (RIA) and radioreceptor assay (RRA). Serumchromatography was performed on Sephadex columns (1×100 cm). The molecular fractions of GH are indicated by the hatched bars, the PRL fraction by open bars. *hGH* human growth hormone, *hPRL* human prolactin

Fig. 3. Growth hormone and prolactin levels in a 40-year-old female patient with a GH- and PRL-producing pituitary tumour after several operations and bromocriptine treatment. Though bromocriptine lowers GH levels in this otherwise therapy-resistant patient, the effect on PRL levels is more pronounced (von Werder K, Fahlbusch R, Landgraf R, Pickardt CR, Rjosk HK, Scriba PC (1978) Treatment of patients with prolactinomas. J Endocrinol Invest 1:47−58). *hGH* human growth hormone, *hPRL* human prolactin, *ACTH* adrenocorticotrophic hormone, *LH* luteinizing hormone, *TSH* thyroid-stimulating hormone

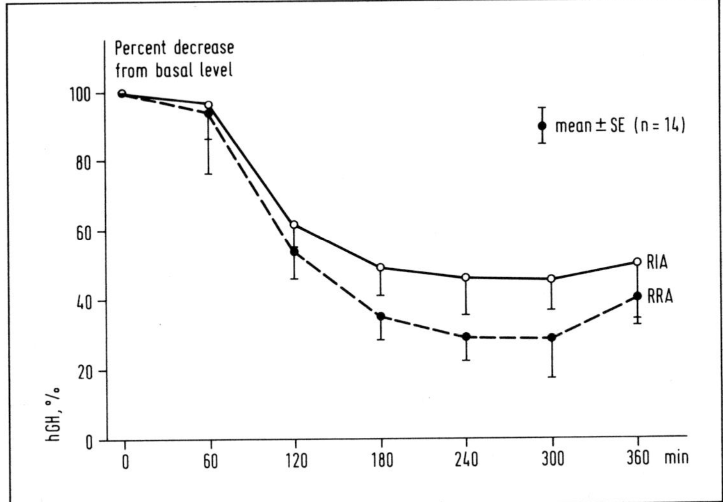

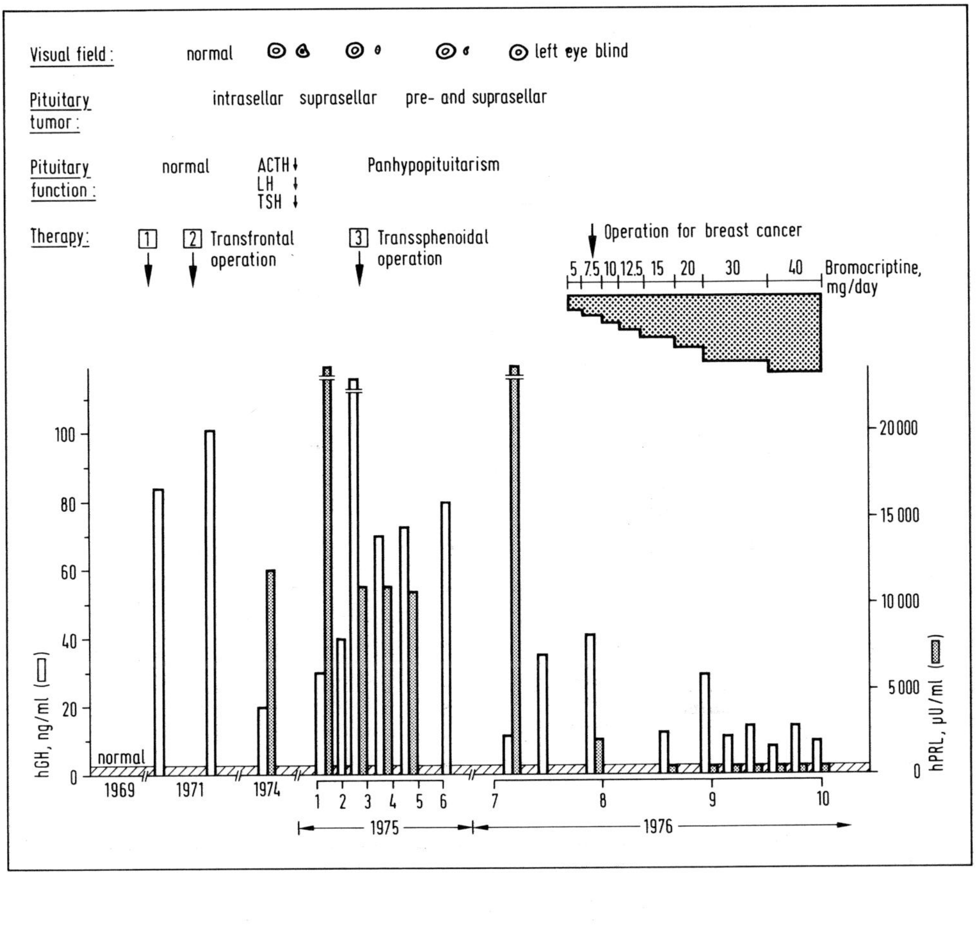

Fig. 2. GH levels measured by radioimmunoassay (RIA) and radioreceptor assay (RRA) in 14 acromegalics after administration of 5 mg bromocriptine p.o. The percentage decrease in radioreceptoractive growth hormone is more pronounced compared with the decrease of radioimmunoassayable GH, though this difference cannot account for the discrepancy between biochemical and clinical improvement observed in bromocriptine-treated acromegalics. *hGH* human growth hormone

erential suppression of monomeric GH leads to a more pronounced fall in the radio-receptor GH activity after bromocriptine ingestion (Fig. 2).

However, these differences are not enough to account for the differences between clinical and biochemical effects of long-term bromocriptine therapy.

Furthermore, Liuzzi et al. [13] could demonstrate a good correlation between GH suppression measured by radioimmunoassay and the fall of the somatomedin-C level induced by dopamine agonist treatment. Since the latter is believed to reflect the clinical activity of the disease [16, 18], the difference between clinical and biochemical improvement of acromegaly remains unexplained.

Though the benefit of bromocriptine treatment in acromegaly has been disputed [11], there is no question that bromocriptine is very useful in the treatment of individual acromegalics. The patient shown in Figure 3 had recurrent acromegaly and hyperprolactinaemia after several operations. She showed definite improvement after long-term bromocriptine therapy had been introduced (Fig. 3).

Another patient had a triple hormone excess with acromegaly, hyperprolactinemia, and ACTH-dependent bilateral adrenal hyperplasia. Again, bromocriptine led to resolution of hyperprolactinaemia, suppression of ACTH levels, and normalization of growth hormone secretion (Fig. 4).

A female patient with hyperprolactinaemia and acromegaly had normal prolactin levels but still elevated growth hormone levels after surgery. Bromocriptine treatment led to a fall in the growth hormone

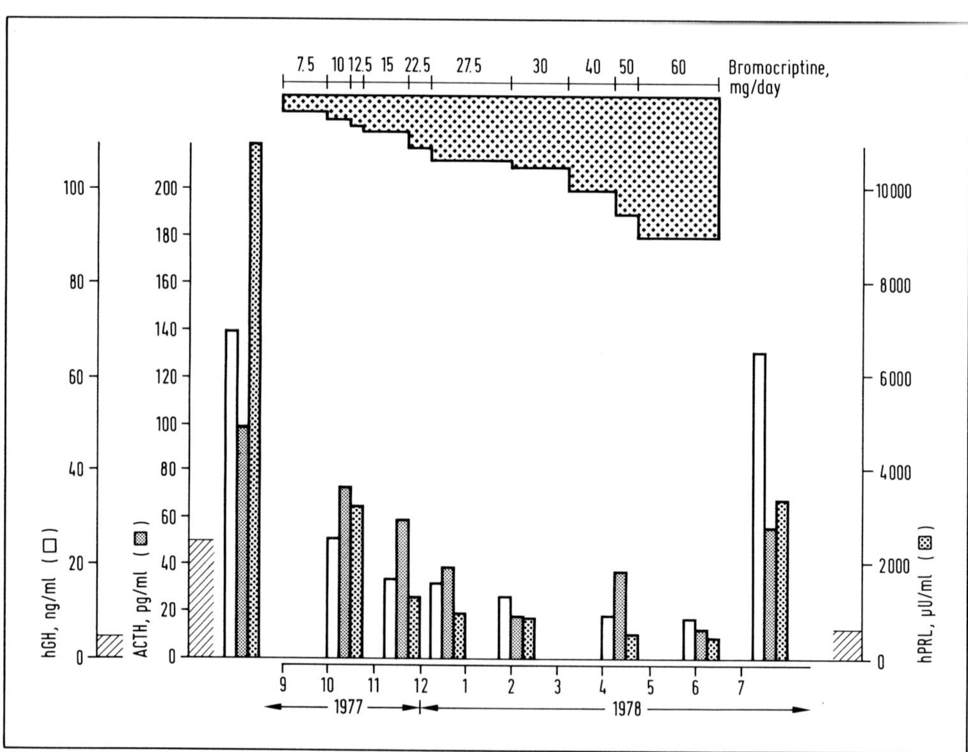

Fig. 4. Growth hormone, ACTH and prolactin levels in a patient with a triple hormone excess. This patient had acromegaly, hyperprolactinaemia, and ACTH-dependent Cushing's disease. Bromocriptine treatment leads to suppression of all 3 hormones. Again the effect on PRL levels is more pronounced compared with the other 2 hormones. Persistent suppression after bromocriptine withdrawal is also only seen with prolactin. *hGH* human growth hormone, *hPRL* human prolactin, *ACTH* adrenocorticotrophic hormone

levels and normalization of the menstrual cycle allowing the patient to become pregnant. Since prolactin levels were normal, the objective improvement of gonadal function must have been induced by the fall in the growth hormone levels.

We have treated altogether 46 patients with bromocriptine for a longer period of time, 41 for persisting GH hypersecretion after surgery and 5 who received primary bromocriptine treatment. The GH levels before treatment ranged from 5 to 798 ng/ml and the bromocriptine dosage ranged from 2.5 to 90 mg/day, the duration of treatment from one to nine years. In 17 patients GH levels under 5 ng/ml were achieved whereas in 9 patients there was a significant fall in the elevated growth hormone levels. In 15 patients no significant effect was seen (Fig. 5). Recurrences with an increase in GH levels were seen in 4 patient during bromocriptine medication; 3 of them developed overt clinical acromegaly again. However, tumour shrinkage has been reported in pure somatotroph tumours [21], Besser has recently claimed that 60% of acromegalic patients showed tumour shrinkage [personal communication]. We have not seen this, which may be due to the fact that the majority of our patients had already undergone

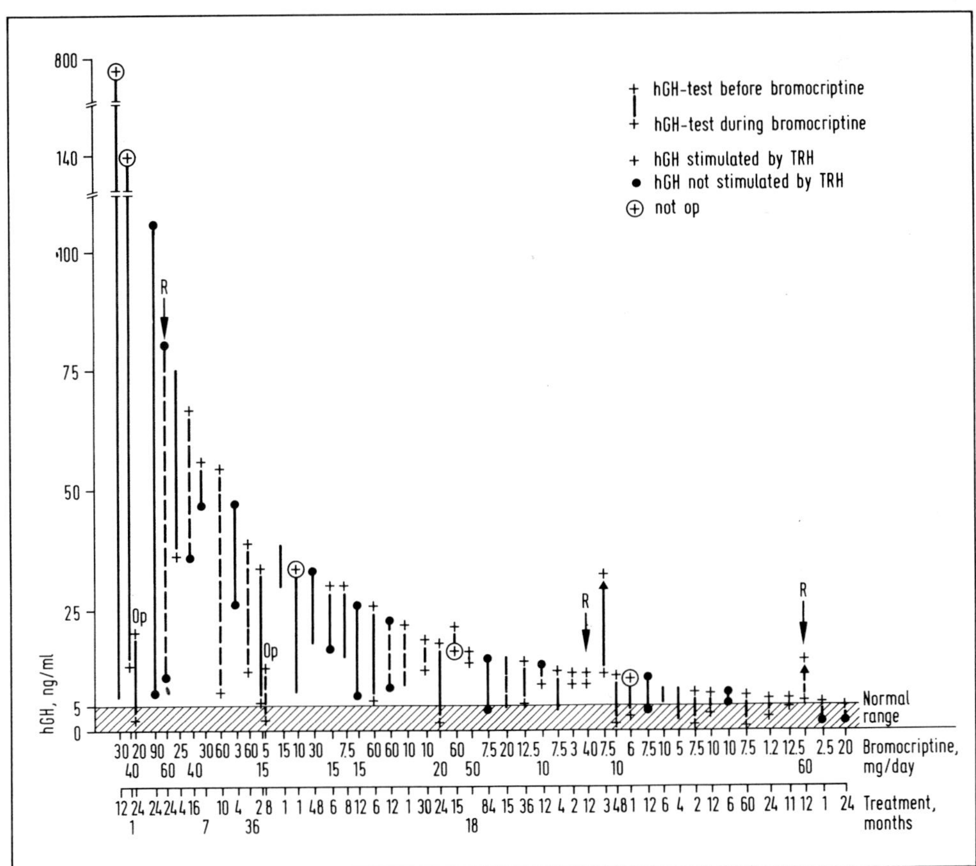

Fig. 5. Growth hormone levels before and during bromocriptine therapy (mean of 3 basal levels) in 46 acromegalic patients. The daily bromocriptine dosage and duration of treatment are shown at the bottom of the figure. The first line of numbers represents the dosage of bromocriptine (mg/day), the bottom line the duration of therapy (months). TRH stimulation of GH secretion (100% increase) is depicted by +. The dashed line represents patients who later received additional therapy, R signals recurrence of active acromegaly [19]. *hGH* human growth hormone, *TRH* thyrotropin releasing hormone

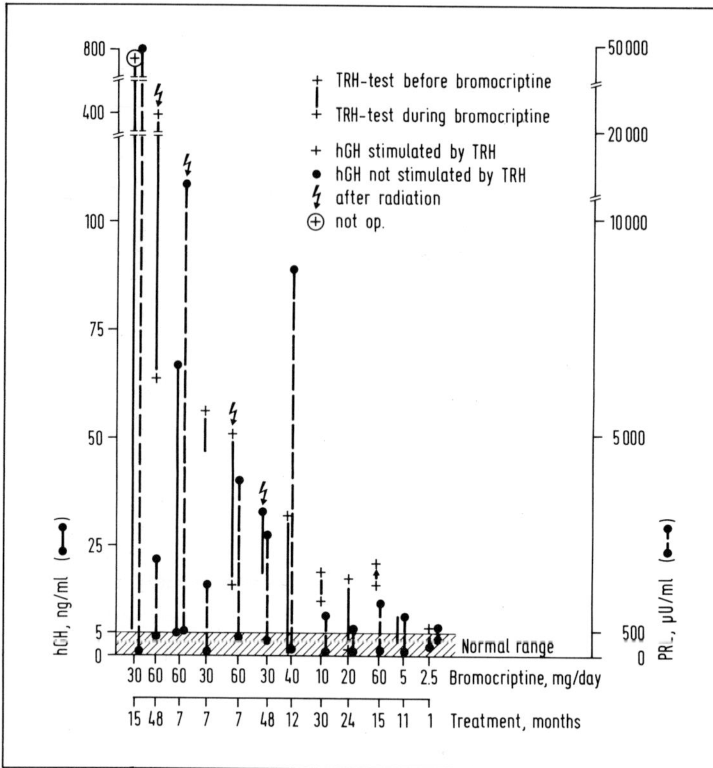

Fig. 6. Growth hormone levels before and during bromocriptine therapy (mean of 3 basal levels) in 12 patients with acromegaly and hyperprolactinaemia. The dosage of bromocriptine and the duration of treatment are shown at the bottom of the Figure. TRH stimulation of GH secretion (100% increase) is depicted by + [19]. *hGH* human growth hormone, *PRL* prolactin, *TRH* thyrotropin releasing hormone

surgery. However, we have seen one patient with a lactotroph somatotroph tumour in whom we observed an increase in tumour volume similar to that reported by other investigators [8]. Though tumour shrinkage seems to occur, the latter is not comparable to the massive shrinkage which is observed in pure lactotroph tumours.

We have also looked at the effect of bromocriptine therapy after previous radiotherapy. Twenty seven patients of whom all had received radiotherapy, 25 after previous surgery, did not respond more markedly than those who had not received radiotherapy, indicating that bromocriptine and radiotherapy have no potentiating effect in lowering growth hormone levels.

Furthermore, 12 patients with acromegaly and hyperprolactinaemia − prolactin levels ranged from 600 to 50 000 µU/ml − received bromocriptine in a dosage of 2.5 to 60 mg/day. Whereas bromocriptine led to normalization of prolactin levels in all 12, GH levels fell below 5 ng/ml only in 5 (Fig. 6). Reduction of GH secretion was seen in 3

whereas no effect upon GH levels was observed in 4 patients. There was no significant increase in the responsiveness of the GH levels to dopaminergic suppression in hyperprolactinaemic acromegalics compared with acromegalics with normal prolactin levels. The TRH/GnRH-stimulated GH secretion was not a prediction of the outcome of long-term dopaminergic therapy, which is in contrast to the short-term results obtained by Lamberts et al. [9].

There is another difference in the effectiveness of bromocriptine when prolactin suppression is compared with growth hormone suppression after long-term treatment with the drug. Whereas prolactin is almost always suppressed, this is not the case in respect of growth hormone and, whereas prolactin remains suppressed for a long period of time after drug withdrawal, growth hormone rises to pretreatment levels immediately when intake of the drug is stopped [19]. How this can be reconciled with the observed tumour shrinkage remains open.

Summary

Table 1. Effect of bromocriptine treatment on serum GH levels in patients with acromegaly

Author(s)	Number of cases	Dosage (mg/day)	Length of treatment (month)	Serum GH levels <5 ng/ml (%)	<10 ng/ml (%)
Besser et al.	101	10–60	9–60	19 (19)	78 (78)
Quabbe	30	10–30	6	10 (33)	23 (78)
Own series	46	2.5–60	10–84	17 (37)	31 (68)

Table 1 summarizes the results obtained with bromocriptine in 3 series of acromegalic patients. It shows that about 25 to 30% of the patients will have GH levels below 5 ng/ml which is a rather poor outcome when compared with the overall results of the surgical treatment [15, 17, 19].

Therefore, though dopamine agonists are effective in patients with growth hormone hypersecretion, they do not represent the first choice treatment [7, 19]. Transsphenoidal surgery or radiotherapy should be performed as an initial step of treatment. However, dopamine agonists are useful in the management of those patients who remain clinically active after the two procedures [19]. Whether the other medical alternative – somatostatin analogues, e.g. Sandostatin® [10] – will make medical therapy of acromegaly a true alternative to surgery or radiotherapy remains to be established.

References

1. Besser GM, Wass JAH, Thorner MO (1980) Bromocriptine in the medical management of acromegaly. Adv Biochem Psychopharmacol 23:191–198
2. Carlson E, Seymour RL, Braunstein GD, Spencer EM, Wilson SE, Hershman JM (1984) Effect of bromocriptine on serum hormones in acromegaly. Horm Res 19: 142–152
3. Chiodini PG, Liuzzi A, Botalla L, Oppizzi G, Müller EE, Silvestrini F (1975) Stable reduction of plasma growth hormone (hGH) levels during chronic administration of 2-Br-ergocryptine (CB-154) in acromegalic patients. J Clin Endocrinol Metab 40:705
4. Daughaday WH (1970) Acromegaly – a stubborn therapeutic challenge. N Engl J Med 282:1430
5. Eastman RC, Gorden P, Roth J (1979) Conventional supervoltage irradiation is an effective treatment for acromegaly. J Clin Endocrinol Metab 48:931
6. Eversmann T, Dietz A, Schopohl J, Gottsmann M, von Werder K (1980) Medikamentöse Therapie der Akromegalie mit Bromocriptin: Immuno- und Rezeptoraktivität des humanen Wachstumshormons. Akt Endokrinol 1:63–72
7. Faglia G, Arosio M, Ambrosi B (1985) Recent advances in diagnosis and treatment of acromegaly. In: Imura H (ed) The pituitary gland. Raven Press, New York, pp 363–404
8. Heidvall K, Hulting A-L (1987) Rapid progression of a growth hormone producing tumour during dopamine agonist treatment. Br Med J 294:346–547
9. Lamberts SWJ, Liuzzi A, Chiodini PG, Verde S, Klijn JGM, Birkenhäger JC (1982) The value of plasma prolactin levels in prediction of the responsiveness of growth hormone secretion to bromocriptine and TRH in acromegaly. Eur J Clin Invest 12:151
10. Lamberts SWJ, Uitterlinden P, Verschoor L, van Dongen KJ, Del Pozo E (1985) Long-term treatment of acromegaly with the somatostatin analogue SMS 201-995. N Engl J Med 313:1576
11. Lindholm J, Riishede J, Vestergaard S, Hummer L, Faber O, Hagen C (1981) No effect of bromocriptine in acromegaly. A controlled trial. N Engl J Med 304:1450–1454
12. Liuzzi A, Chiodini PG, Botalla L, Cremascoli G, Silvestrini F (1972) Inhibitory effect of L-dopa on GH-release in acromegalic patients. J Clin Endocrinol Metab 35:941
13. Liuzzi A, Chiodini PG, Cozzi R, Dallabonzana D, Oppizzi G, Petroncini M, Verde G (1987) The medical treatment of acromegaly with Lisuride and its derivates. In: Lüdecke DK, Tolis G (eds) Growth hormone, growth factors, and acromegaly. Raven Press, New York, pp 189–198
14. Losa M, Schopohl J, Müller OA, von Werder

K (1985) Growth hormone releasing factor induces prolactin secretion in acromegalic patients but not in normal subjects. Acta Endocrinol (Copenh) 109:467

15. Lüdecke DK (1985) Recent development in the treatment of acromegaly. Neurosurg Rev 8:167

16. Melmed S, Braunstein GD, Horváth E, Ezrin C, Kovács K (1983) Pathophysiology of acromegaly. Endocr Rev 4:271

17. Quabbe H-J (1982) Treatment of acromegaly by transsphenoidal operation, 90-Yttrium implantation and bromocriptine: results in 230 patients. Clin Endocrinol 16:107

18. Schaison G, Couzinet B, Moatti N, Pertuiset B (1983) Critical study of the growth hormone response to dynamic tests and the insulin growth factor assay in acromegaly after microsurgery. Clin Endocrinol 18:541

19. von Werder K, Eversmann T, Losa M, Oeckler R, Pichl J, Fahlbusch R (1987) Decision analysis of treatment options in acromegaly. In: Robbins R, Melmed S (eds) Acromegaly. A century of scientific and clinical progress. Plenum Press, New York London, pp 267–280

20. Wass JAM, Clemmons DR, Underwood LE, Barrow I, Besser GM, Van Wyk JJ (1982) Changes in circulating somatomedin-C levels in bromocriptine-treated acromegaly. Clin Endocrinol (Oxf) 17:369

21. Wass JAM, Moult PJA, Thorner MO, Dacie JE, Charlesworth M, Jones AE, Besser GM (1979) Reduction in pituitary tumour size in patients with prolactinomas and acromegaly treated with bromocriptine with or without radiotherapy. Lancet II:66

7. Chemical Structure, Pharmacodynamic Profile and Pharmacokinetics of SMS 201-995 (Sandostatin®)

P. Marbach[1], H. Andres[2], M. Azria[2], W. Bauer[1], U. Briner[1], K.-H. Buchheit[1], W. Doepfner[1], M. Lemaire[2], T. J. Petcher[1], J. Pless[1], J.-C. Reubi[1]

Preclinical Research Department[1] and Pharmaceutical Development Department[2], Sandoz Ltd, Basle, Switzerland

Natural somatostatin (SRIF) is a tetradecapeptide with a multiplicity of inhibiting actions on the secretion of a variety of hormones. *In vivo,* the compound has a biological half-life of only two to three minutes and its clinical route of application is therefore restricted to that of intravenous infusion. The challenge facing peptide chemists over the last one and a half decades has been on the one hand to increase the stability of the molecule and thus improve the duration of action, and on the other to design analogues with an improved specificity in respect of selective inhibition of the secretion of a single hormone.

Drug Design

J. Rivier performed elegant work at the Salk Institute in a resolute pursuit of the "minimal essential sequence" of SRIF (Table 1), in the course of which he synthesized a number of analogues of reduced size. This work led to the conclusion that, while the sequence Phe^6 to Phe^{11} is important for reasonable biological activity, the sequence Phe^7 to Thr^{10} is essential.

In our laboratories, the strategy adopted to obtain highly active analogues with a reduced size was the stepwise incorporation of additional structural elements of the natural tetradecapeptide into this minimal essential sequence. The tetrapeptide sequence Phe^7 to Thr^{10} was first conformationally stabilized by means of cyclization with a cys-

Table 1. Biological potencies of $[D\text{-}Trp^8]$-oligosomatostatins. In vitro activity was determined in primary cell cultures of rat pituitaries. (Data taken from Vale et al. [6])

AAS deleted	No. AA	Structure	GH in vitro (SRIF = 100)
–	14	Ala-Gly-Cys-Lys-Asn-Phe-Phe-DTrp Cys - Ser - Thr - Phe - Thr - Lys	800
1,2	12	Cys-Lys-Ans-Phe-Phe-DTrp Cys - Ser - Thr - Phe - Thr - Lys	400
1,2,4,5	10	Cys————Phe - Phe - DTrp Cys - Ser - Thr - Phe - Thr - Lys	110
1,2,4,5,12,13	8	Cys————Phe - Phe - DTrp Cys————Phe - Thr - Lys	4
1,2,4,5,11,12,13	7	Cys————Phe - Phe - DTrp Cys————Thr - Lys	0.07

Table 2. Structures and biological activities of SRIF analogues (A-Cys-Phe-DTrp-Lys-Thr-Cys-B). *In vitro* activities were measured in primary cell cultures of rat pituitaries after stimulation with isobutyl-methylxanthine (IBMX). Cells were cultured for 4 days, incubation with peptides was for 3 h. *In vivo* potencies were determined 15 min after i.m. administration in male rats under Nembutal anaesthesia. SMS is the abbreviation for Sandostatin

| | Substituents | | Potency GH (SRIF = 100) | |
	A	B	in vitro	in vivo
1	H	NH$_2$	<0.1	1.4
2	H	D-Ser(NH$_2$)	<0.1	3.3
3	D-Phe	NH$_2$	4	165
4	D-Phe	D-Ser(NH$_2$)	12	680
5	D-Phe	Ser(ol)	19	2800
6	D-Phe	Phe(ol)	32	650
7	D-Phe	D-Thr(NH$_2$)	47	1160
8	D-Phe	D-Thr(ol)	54	1100
SMS	D-Phe	L-Thr(ol)	300	7000

tine bridge (Table 2). Physical and computer-assisted model building suggested that D-Phe at the amino-terminal end might be able to occupy at least part of the conformational space available to Phe[6] of SRIF. Compound 3 was the first to show reasonable biological activity in our cell culture system. Further addition of structural elements at the carboxyl-terminal position enhanced activity both *in vitro* and *in vivo*. Compound 9, with the code name SMS 201-995, represented the culmination of this strategy and was selected for further development.

It is of interest that the *in vitro* activity of this compound is not particularly high when compared with SRIF, but the *in vivo* activity is outstanding. This may be taken as evidence that the most important improvement achieved in relation to natural SRIF is high stability against metabolic degradation, which has led to a favourable pharmacokinetic profile. Molecular modelling techniques show that SMS 201-995 almost perfectly mimics that fragment of SRIF which had been identified as being essential for biological activity [1,7].

Pharmacodynamic Profile

Potency and Duration of Action

The following four experiments, selected from the many we have performed, will serve to demonstrate the high biological potency of Sandostatin® (SMS 201-995).

Experiment 1: Conscious rats with chronically implanted catheters in the jugular vein received subcutaneous injections of Sandostatin. Every fifteen minutes, morphine was infused through the catheter in order to stimulate the secretion of growth hormone (GH), and blood was sampled immediately before each morphine dose. GH levels were measured by means of specific radioimmunoassay (RIA) and expressed in percent of the control group (Fig. 1). It is evident that Sandostatin inhibited GH secretion to the same extent as SRIF, and for a significantly longer time, at doses which were one thousand times lower than those of SRIF.

Experiment 2: SRIF and Sandostatin were injected subcutaneously in pentobarbital-anaesthetized rats. After different intervals of time, the rats were decapitated, trunk blood was collected, and GH levels were measured by means of RIA. Fifteen minutes after the administration of the drugs, the ED$_{50}$ for inhibition of GH secretion were 8.2 µg/kg and 0.08 µg/kg for SRIF and for Sandostatin respectively. After one hour, this potency ratio had increased from 100 to 12 000. Six hours after administration, Sandostatin was still half as potent as was SRIF 15 min after administration.

The experiments described above demonstrate rather dramatically that Sandostatin has a longer duration of action than SRIF; and that the potency ratio is both very

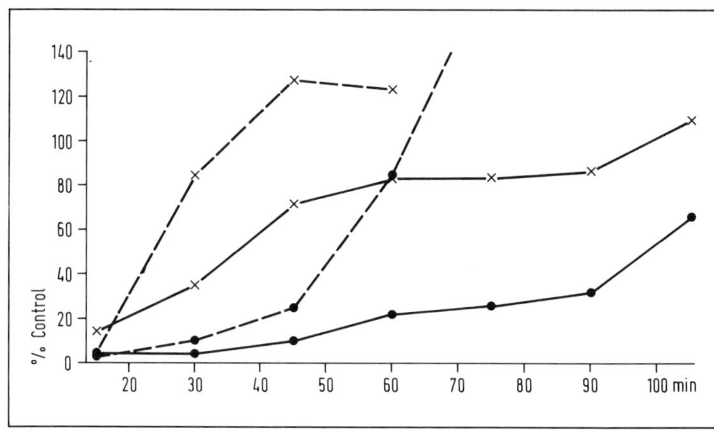

Fig. 1. Time and dose-dependent effects on morphine-stimulated growth hormone secretion in the rat. Sandostatin (solid lines) was given at doses of 0.1 µg/kg s.c. (×) and 1 µg/kg s.c. (●) and somatostatin (broken lines) in doses of 100 µg/kg s.c. (×) and 1000 µg/kg s.c. (●) respectively. Morphine 1 mg/kg was injected i.v. every 15 min, immediately after blood sampling. (N = 7 per dose)

high and dependent on the experimental conditions. The following two examples show that the very high potency and stability of Sandostatin result in oral activity after application of a reasonable dose in different animal species.

Experiment 3: Male rats were implanted with gastric fistulae. After a recovery period of at least seven days, experiments were commenced by starving the animals for 18 h. Either Sandostatin or cimetidine was given orally in water. One hour after drug administration, i.e. after that time which had previously been determined to be necessary for complete clearance of the given volume from the stomach, the fistula was opened and the gastric juice sampled half-hourly. Figure 2 clearly shows that 0.5 mg/kg Sandostatin was equi-active to 10 mg/kg cimetidine with regard to both potency and duration of action.

No difference was seen in the qualitative effects; neither drug affected either the concentration of bound acid or the volume of

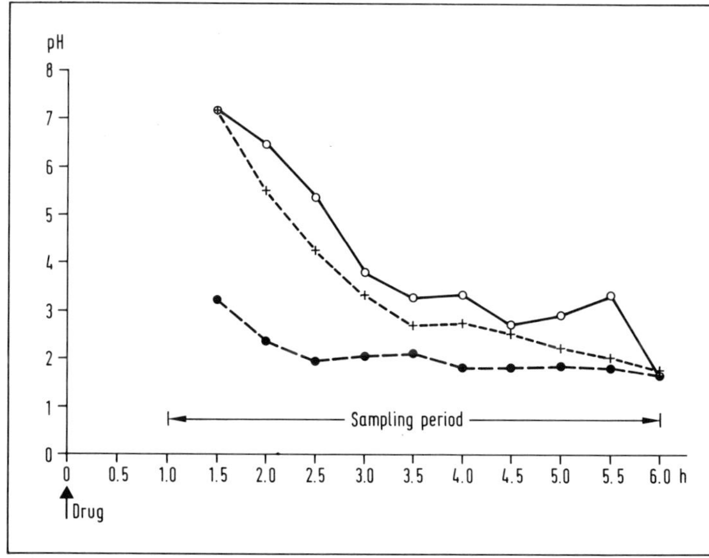

Fig. 2. Oral administration of Sandostatin and cimetidine in the rat: effects on gastric acid secretion. Sandostatin (×) 0.5 mg/kg and cimetidine (○) 10 mg/kg were applied orally at time zero and the effect on the pH of the secreted gastric juice was compared with control rats (●). N = 5 per dose. Note that an increase of 1 pH unit indicates 90% reduction of acid concentration

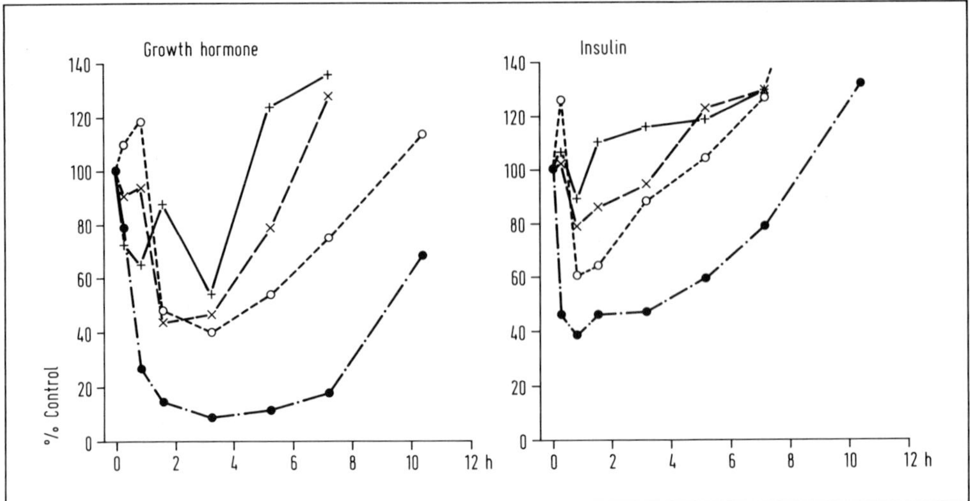

Fig. 3. Oral application of Sandostatin in the rhesus monkey: effects on growth hormone and insulin. Sandostatin was given together with a small piece of banana in doses of 0.01 (+), 0.03 (×), 0.1 (○), and 1 (●) mg/kg respectively. The results are expressed in percent of control values after the application of placebo, in this case a small piece of banana. (N = 4−7 per dose, 12 in the control group)

juice secreted. These results show, together with the known inhibitory effect of somatostatin on the secretion of gastrin [2], a profile of action for Sandostatin which suggests its potential applicability in peptic ulcer disease [3].

Experiment 4: Male rhesus monkeys were adapted to a chair and to sitting in it for the duration of the experiment. Drugs were given orally together with a small piece of banana. Blood sampling was performed in an essentially stress-free manner from an adjacent room via a catheter chronically implanted in the saphenous vein. The animals were fasted overnight prior to each experiment. Figure 3 shows the effects of Sandostatin on the secretion of growth hormone and of insulin. The inhibition of secretion was dose-dependent and long-lasting. Natural somatostatin inhibited the secretion of GH and insulin by 75% after a dose of 0.1 mg/kg subcutaneously, but this effect was transient and lasted only 30 min (data not shown). It can be seen that the effect of Sandostatin upon insulin secretion was of much shorter duration than on GH secretion. Thus the specificity of Sandostatin in inhibiting GH, rather than insulin, secretion is a time-dependent phenomenon.

Specificity

Somatostatin was first described as a growth hormone release-inhibiting factor. It soon became clear, however, that SRIF has a multiplicity of inhibitory activities, for example on the secretion of insulin, glucagon, gastrin, thyroid-stimulating hormone, and a variety of peptide hormones of gastrointestinal origin. It was therefore an important goal of analogue design to synthesize peptides with more specific actions. The inhibitory effect on insulin secretion was regarded by us as representing the principal disadvantage for potential long-term administration in indications such as acromegaly and especially non-insulin-dependent diabetes mellitus.

When we looked at the actions of Sandostatin on GH, insulin, and glucagon secretion in the rat, we found that relative to SRIF, the analogue was 70 times more potent in its action on the release of GH, but only 3 times more potent on the release of insulin. Sandostatin thus had an improved selectivity for GH in relation to insulin by a factor of 70 to 3, i.e. 23. These hormone measurements were all performed 15 min after intramuscular administration of the drug. After subcutaneous administration in

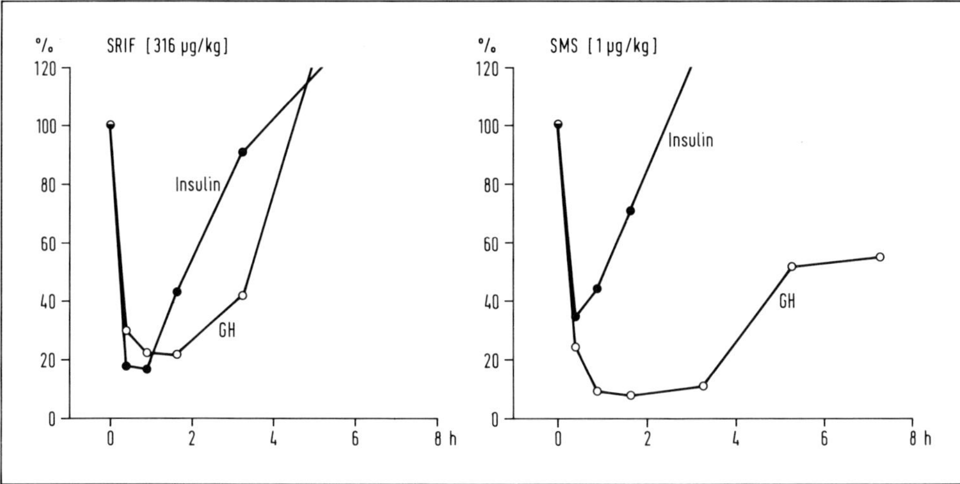

Fig. 4. Specific effects of somatostatin and Sandostatin in monkeys after s.c. administration in the thigh. SRIF was given at a dose of 316 µg/kg and Sandostatin at a dose of 1 µg/kg. GH (○) and insulin (●) were determined by means of RIA. *GH* growth hormone

the conscious male rhesus monkey (Fig. 4) it became clearly apparent that the measured specificity is mainly a reflection of the different time courses of action of the drug on the secretion of different hormones, the effect on GH being much more prolonged. Even with SRIF, the effect on GH relative to insulin secretion is stronger to a slight but significant degree, but Sandostatin showed a much more favourable profile − a dose of 1 µg/kg s.c. had a less potent effect than 316 µg/kg SRIF on insulin secretion but a more potent effect on GH secretion.

Tumour Models

There are many reasons why it would be of interest to mimic human diseases in animal models. In this short overview of the pharmacology of Sandostatin we will confine ourselves to two examples. In receptor binding studies, high-affinity binding sites for SRIF can be demonstrated both on pituitary cells and in the pancreas [4]. It is therefore reasonable to expect receptor-mediated effects of somatostatin in these two organs.

Estrogen-Induced Pituitary Hyperplasia

When rats are implanted with a Silastic®

tube containing estradiol (E2), they develop hyperplasia of the pituitary gland and marked hyperprolactinaemia. The specific concentration of prolactin-mRNA increases whereas that of GH-mRNA diminishes. In contrast to its effects in normal rats, Sandostatin potently inhibits the secretion of prolactin in E2-treated rats. This could be shown both *in vitro* (data not shown) and *in vivo*.

In a typical experiment, male rats were implanted with 10 mg E2. After two months, they were divided into different groups. The control group continued to receive E2 from the implant, but no other treatment. The second group received in addition 10 µg/kg/h Sandostatin from a subcutaneously implanted Alzet minipump. The third group had their E2 implants removed. In these latter rats, the E2 concentration in blood fell from 260 pg/ml to normal levels of about 6 pg/ml within one day. The established pituitary hyperplasia was reduced by 50% within a month and the elevated prolactin levels returned to normal within one to two weeks. In the Sandostatin-treated group, pituitary size was reduced by 35% after one month and prolactin levels were decreased by 65%. In the control group, the already increased pituitary size remained constant or even tended to further increase. This effect of Sandostatin might be of relevance for the treatment of estrogen-dependent neoplasias.

Insulinoma

Fragments of a hamster insulinoma bearing high-affinity somatostatin receptors were freshly transplanted in hamsters. The animals were then treated daily with 200 µg/kg Sandostatin subcutaneously. After one month, tumour growth was inhibited by 40% compared with controls. A moderate effect of Sandostatin on the growth of well-established insulinomas could thus be observed [5]. This effect may be of relevance for the use of Sandostatin in the treatment of gastroenteropancreatic tumours.

Pharmacokinetics

Disposition in the Rat

Pharmacokinetic parameters were measured by means of three tools. First, the development of a specific radioimmunoassay for Sandostatin enabled us to determine precisely the concentration of unchanged peptide in plasma and in various tissues. Second, a tritiated form of the molecule was synthesized in which the radioactive isotope was introduced into the side chain of the lysine residue. Third, an alternative radio-labelling was performed by introduction of ^{14}C into the side chain of the D-tryptophan. Similar plasma levels and excretion values were obtained using the three different analytical techniques. Sandostatin exhibits a markedly prolonged half-life of 20 min in plasma after s.c. injection, which compares favourably with the 2−3 min observed for SRIF. When administered s.c. and i.v. to bile-duct-cannulated rats, 50% and 73% of the given dose respectively were excreted in bile within eight hours, essentially as unchanged drug. About 20 to 25% of the administered dose appeared in the urine, again unmetabolized. In intact animals, almost no unchanged drug could be recovered from the faeces. It can be concluded from these results that Sandostatin is extremely stable in the circulation, is mainly excreted via the bile, and is then broken down by the

local fauna in its further passage through the intestinal tract. Figure 5 shows representative HPLC profiles of the radioactivity in various biological fluids and in the faeces

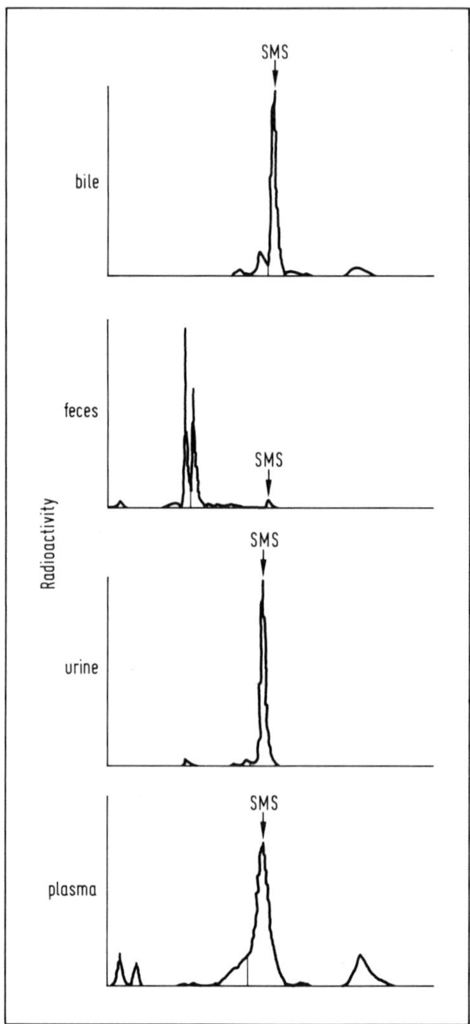

Fig. 5. HPLC-chromatograms after i.v. administration of ^{14}C-labelled Sandostatin (SMS) in the rat. Chromatograms were run on RP-18 columns, 0.46 × 10 cm, equipped with a pre-column. The elution gradient was from 0 to 10% (2 min), 10 to 20% (5 min), and 20 to 65% (25 min) solvent B in A respectively at a flow rate of 1.5 ml/min. Solvent A: 0.2% TFA in water, solvent B: 0.2% TFA in acetonitrile. Bile, urine, and faeces were pooled samples from 0 to 2, 7, and 24 h respectively; plasma was taken at 30 min after administration

after intravenous administration of Sandostatin in the rat.

Organ Distribution Pattern

In order to study further the distribution of Sandostatin, the concentrations of the drug in different organs were determined. Sandostatin was administered subcutaneously to rats at a dose of 1 mg/kg. At different intervals, the animals were killed and their organs dissected out and homogenized in acidic methanol. The extracts were lyophilized in a Speed-Vac concentrator and taken up in buffer for determination of drug concentrations by means of RIA. The recovery rate of this procedure was greater than 80%. Thirty minutes after the administration of Sandostatin, unchanged drug amounted to 517 ng/ml in the plasma, 345 pg/mg in the skin (excepting the site of injection), 94 pg/mg in the pancreas, and 98 pg/mg in the pituitary. Seven hours after administration, drug levels were 1.2 ng/ml and 26, 127, and 60 pg/mg respectively. These data highlight the differences in pharmacokinetic behaviour in assumed target and non-target organs. The very slow elimination from presumed target organs may partially explain the long duration of action of Sandostatin, particularly after subcutaneous injection.

Safety

Sandostatin was extremely well tolerated after single application in various species. In the primary observation test in rats, where effects both on the central nervous system and on the periphery are closely monitored, and in cardiovascular investigations in the cat, Sandostatin showed no untoward side effects. In particular, there was no respiratory disturbance, no appearance of stereotyped behaviour, and no changes in muscle tone even with doses of 3 mg/kg s.c. Doses several orders of magnitude higher than those which elicited endocrine effects produced only a minor reduction in blood pressure and a slight potentiation of the pressor effects of noradrenalin.

In a 26-week intraperitoneal study in rats, Sandostatin was well tolerated at doses of 0.02, 0.1 and 1 mg/kg/day. Histological examination revealed no changes attributable to drug treatment. The no-toxic-effect level (NTEL) could be set at 1 mg/kg/day, which gives a safety factor of approximately 150 to 1500 when compared with the doses intended for administration in various indications in man.

Summary

Sandostatin is an analogue of SRIF with dramatically improved biological stability. This has led to a considerable increase in duration of action, which circumvents the necessity for intravenous infusion – the analogue may conveniently be administered by subcutaneous injection. The prolonged biological half-life further elicits a marked specificity for inhibition of the secretion of growth hormone, since the inhibitory effect on insulin secretion is much shorter-lived, probably because of counter-regulatory mechanisms. It has been possible to demonstrate a beneficial effect of Sandostatin on the growth of tumours.

Pharmacokinetic measurements demonstrate the stability of Sandostatin in biological fluids and in tissues and reveal a high biliary excretion together with a slow rate of disappearance from target tissues.

All these favourable properties, taken together with the lack of important side effects after acute and long-term administration, make Sandostatin a very attractive potential drug for the treatment of acromegaly, gastroenteropancreatic tumours, hypersecretory disorders of the gastrointestinal tract, and of diabetes.

References

1. Bauer W, Briner U, Doepfner W, Haller R, Huguenin R, Marbach P, Petcher TJ, Pless J (1982) SMS 201–995: A very potent and selective octapeptide analogue of somatostatin with prolonged action. Life Sci 31:1133–1140
2. Bloom SR, Mortimer Ch, Thorner MO, Besser GM, Hall R, Gomez-Pan A, Roy VM, Russel RCG, Coy DH, Kastin AJ, Schally AV (1974) Inhibition of gastrin and gastric acid secretion by growth hormone release inhibiting hormone. Lancet II:1106–1109

3. Kayesseh L, Gyr K, Keller U, Stalder GA, Wall M (1980) Somatostatin and cimetidine in peptic-ulcer haemorrhage. Lancet i: 844−846
4. Reubi JC (1984) Evidence for two somatostatin-14 receptor types in rat brain cortex. Neurosci Lett 49:259−263
5. Reubi JC (1985) A somatostatin analogue inhibits chondrosarcoma and insulinoma tumour growth. Acta Endocrinol 109: 108−114
6. Vale W, Rivier J, Ling N, Brown M (1978) Biologic and immunologic activities and applications of somatostatin analogues. Metabolism 27:1391−1401
7. Wynants C, van Binst G, Loosli HR (1985) SMS 201-995, a very potent analogue of somatostatin; assignment of the ^{1}H 500 MHz n.m.r. spectra and conformational analysis in aqueous solution. Int J Pept Protein Res 25:608−614

8. Studies on the Acute and Chronic Effects of Sandostatin® in Acromegaly

S. W. J. Lamberts

Department of Medicine, Erasmus University, Rotterdam, The Netherlands

The hypothalamic hormones, somatostatin and growth hormone releasing hormone (GHRH) play a central role in the regulation of normal growth hormone (GH) secretion. Studies using cultured tumor cells prepared from the GH-secreting pituitary adenomas of acromegalic patients, showed that hormone secretion by these cells has retained qualitatively a high sensitivity to the inhibitory effect of somatostatin and to the stimulatory effect of GHRH [10]. On a molar base, somatostatin inhibits GHRH-stimulated GH secretion by these cultured human pituitary tumor cells in a non-competitive manner, making somatostatin in theory an excellent drug for the treatment of acromegaly. It took many years after the initial discovery of somatostatin [3] to prepare a clinically useful long-acting somatostatin analog which has proved to be successful in the chronic treatment of this disease. Sandostatin® (octreotide, SMS 201-995) is a preferentially GH-inhibitory analog of somatostatin, which can be administered subcutaneously or even orally [25] and has a half-life after subcutaneous administration of 113 min [2, 7].

The Acute Effects of Sandostatin

A typical example of the effects of Sandostatin on circulating GH, glucose and insulin levels is shown in Figure 1. In this acromegalic patient mean GH levels amounted on a control day to 36 ± 3 µg/l (mean ± SEM; n = 17 samples collected over 24 h). The subcutaneous administration of 25, 50 and 100 µg Sandostatin induced a rapid and impressive inhibition of the plasma GH concentrations, which was maximal 2 h after administration of the drug. The effect of these

three doses of Sandostatin on GH secretion differed especially with regard to the duration of the inhibitory effect on GH release. In other, more extensive, studies in 7 acromegalic patients [9], we showed that 50 and 100 µg Sandostatin induced, from 2 to 6 h after subcutaneous administration, a similar reduction of GH levels by 85% and 86%, respectively. However, the dose of 100 µg Sandostatin caused a significantly longer inhibitory effect on GH than did 50 µg: from 2 to 10 h after administration of the drug GH levels were suppressed by 62% after 50 µg and by 81% after 100 µg Sandostatin (p < 0.01).

The postprandial increment of glucose after breakfast increased in a dose-dependent manner after Sandostatin administration (Fig. 1, middle part). This was caused by a short-lived dose-dependent inhibition of insulin secretion for only about 2 h. Earlier studies in normal volunteers showed that Sandostatin inhibits normal GH and insulin secretion for about 3.5–4 and 1.5–2 h, respectively [7]. Therefore it can be concluded from Figure 1 that the somatostatin analog exerts a much longer inhibitory effect on tumoral than on normal GH secretion, making it a very attractive drug for the chronic treatment of acromegaly. Further, of paramount importance is the absence of a rebound hypersecretion of hormones as the effect of the drug tapers off; this, in sharp contrast to the rebound hypersecretion observed after the intravenous administration of natural somatostatin [11].

We investigated the acute effect of the subcutaneous injection of 50 µg Sandostatin on plasma GH levels in comparison with the hormone levels on a control day in 41 consecutive acromegalic patients. Mean plasma GH levels were 42 ± 11 µg/l on a control day

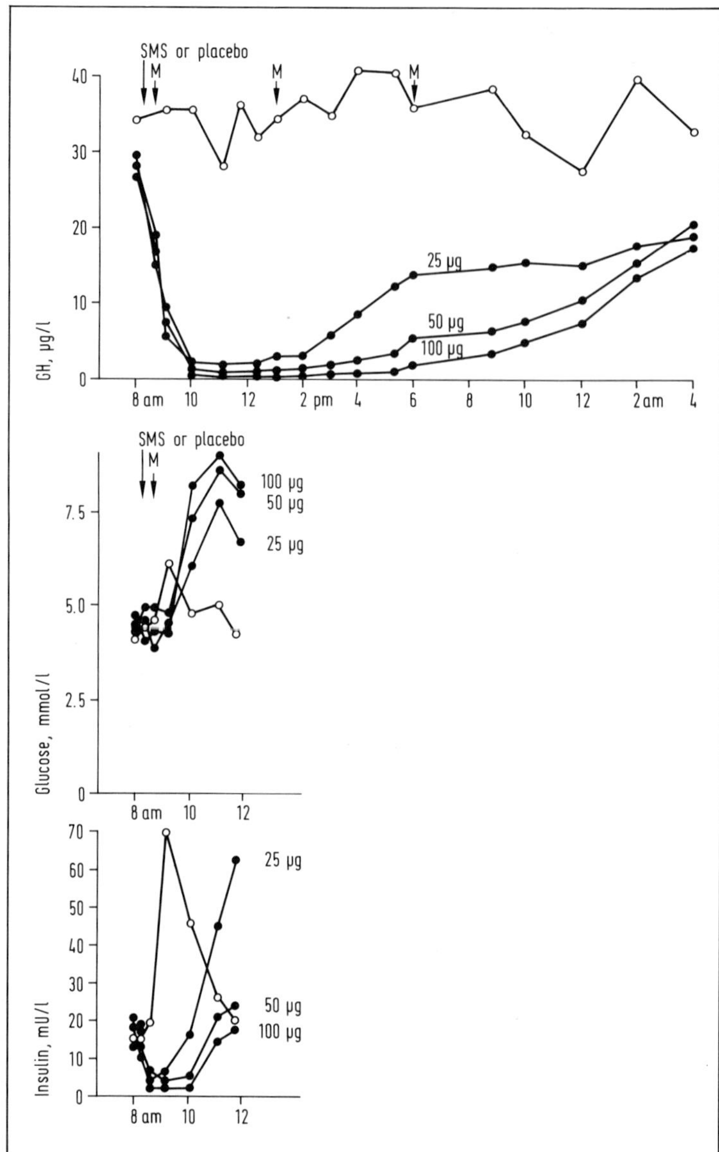

Fig. 1. A comparison between the effects of the subcutaneous administration of 25, 50 and 100 µg Sandostatin (SMS) (●—●) and of placebo (○—○) on plasma growth hormone (GH), glucose and insulin levels in a 56-year-old untreated male acromegalic patient. M = meal. (With kind permission from [9])

but were suppressed to 8 ± 2 µg/l (−81 ± 4%) from 2 to 6 h after Sandostatin administration (Fig. 2). The plasma GH concentrations were suppressed to below 5 µg/l in 24 (58%) of these 41 patients and to below 50% of the levels on the control day in 34 (83%) of them. These data point to a considerable variation in the sensitivity to Sandostatin of GH secretion in acromegalic patients. GH secretion in 17% of these pa-

tients shows a rather low sensitivity to somatostatin. This observation is closely parallel to the studies by Reubi and Landolt [24] who showed a considerable variation in the number of somatostatin receptors on the pituitary tumors of acromegalic patients.

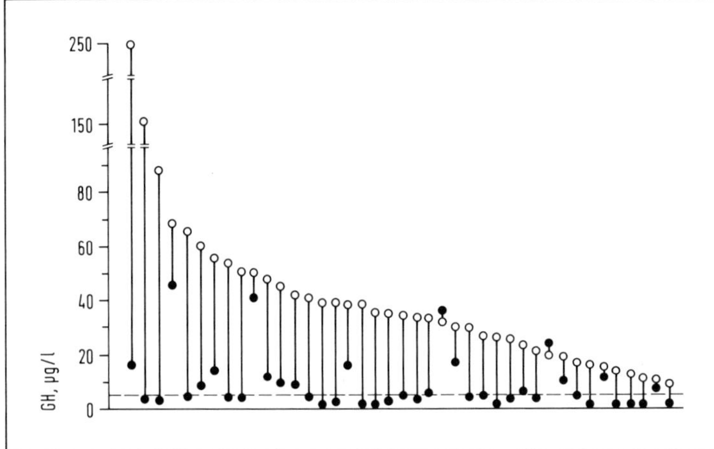

Fig. 2. The effect of 50 µg Sandostatin in 41 acromegalic patients on mean plasma growth hormone (GH) concentrations 2–6 h after injection (● = mean of 5 samples) in comparison with those on a control day (○)

Chronic Treatment

Several reports have been published so far which show that acromegalic patients respond favorably to chronic treatment with Sandostatin [1, 4, 5, 8, 12, 20–23]. Our own results involving chronic treatment for a mean of 66 weeks of 10 patients with Sandostatin in a dose of 200–300 µg daily in two or three subcutaneous injections were recently published [16].

In all 10 patients long-term Sandostatin treatment resulted in rapid clinical improvement that ranged from modest to complete disappearance of signs and symptoms. Excessive sweating, headache, paresthesias and tiredness markedly decreased within the first weeks of treatment and disappeared during long-term treatment in most patients (Fig. 3). A decrease in soft tissue swelling and remodelling and improvement of the classical features of acromegaly were

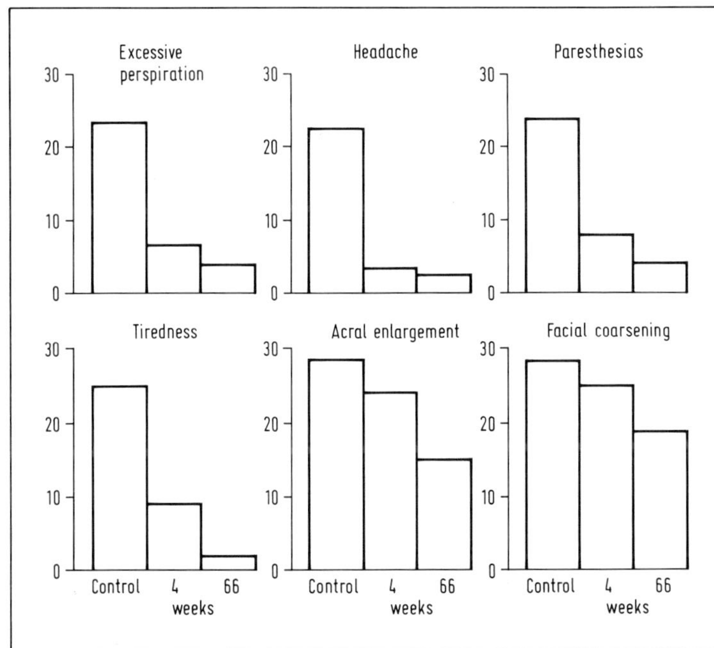

Fig. 3. Course of clinical features before (left column), after 4 (middle column), and after 66 weeks (right column) of treatment with Sandostatin (300 µg/day) of 10 acromegalic patients. Values indicate cumulative data according to an arbitrary scale between 0 (absent) and 3 (severe)

noted in all patients after longer periods of treatment.

Each subcutaneous administration of Sandostatin was followed by a rapid decline in circulating GH levels in all patients, in most instances for several hours, to below 5 µg/l or even to be undetectable. However, 5−7 h after drug administration the GH levels gradually increased again in all patients towards the next injection (Fig. 4). This tendency to increase remained evident in most patients even after 2 years of Sandostatin therapy. However, chronic continuous therapy with three injections of the drug per day resulted in a gradual decrease in this tendency of GH levels to increase towards the next injection. Typical 24-h GH profiles during long-term Sandostatin treatment from a patient in whom a gradual further decrease of the mean GH levels occurred is shown in Figure 5. It is evident that the serum somatomedin-C (Sm-C) levels in this patient also gradually further decreased parallel to the mean GH levels; the Sm-C value eventually normalized in this patient after 2 years of Sandostatin therapy (Fig. 5, lower part). In a total of 6 patients in whom the 24-h GH profiles and Sm-C levels could

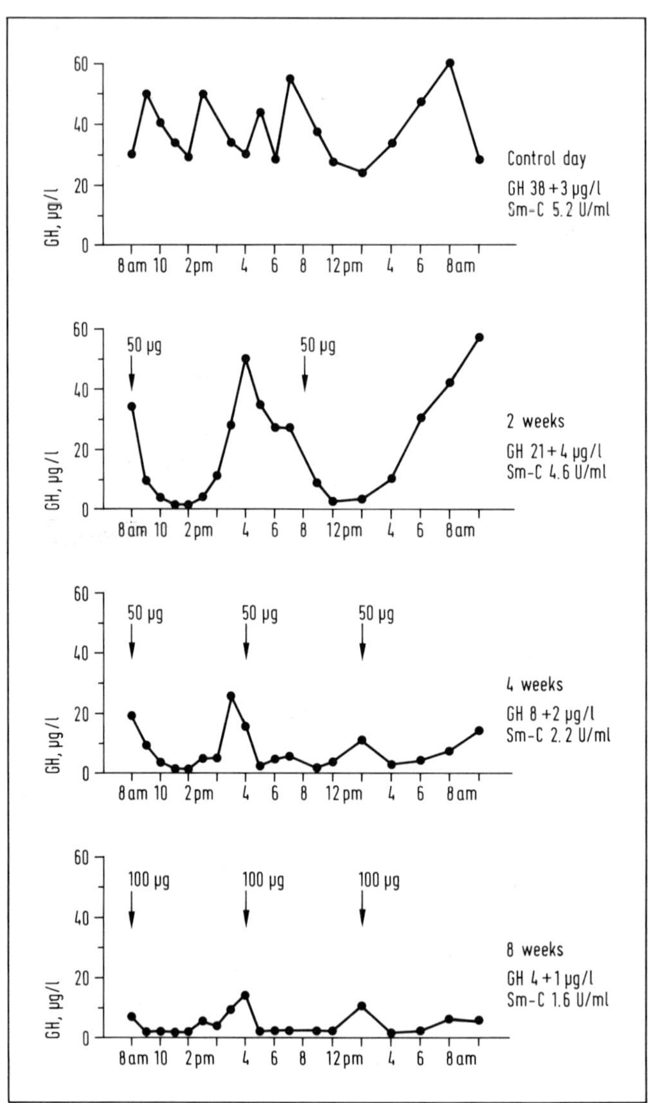

Fig. 4. The effect of various doses of Sandostatin on plasma growth hormone (GH) profiles over 24 h and on somatomedin-C (Sm-C) levels in a 36-year-old male acromegalic. (With kind permission from [11])

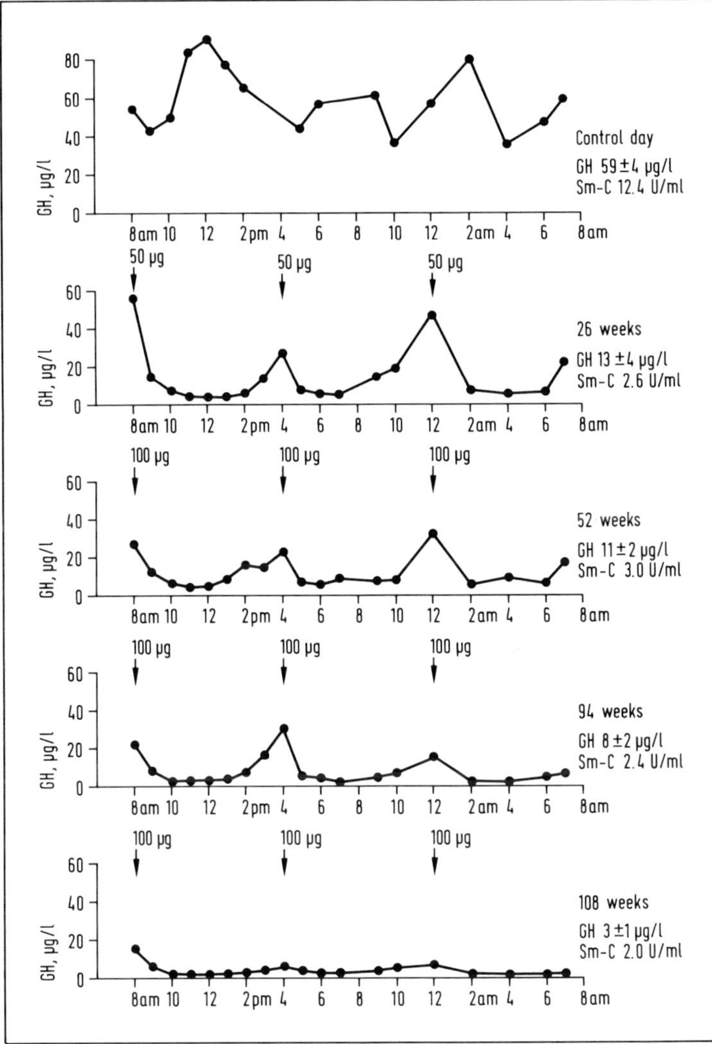

Fig. 5. The effect of long-term therapy with Sandostatin on plasma growth hormone (GH) profiles and on somatomedin-C (Sm-C) levels in a 37-year-old male acromegalic. (With kind permission from [16])

be regularly measured during long-term therapy with 200–300 µg/day for 1.5–2 years, this slow, gradual, further improvement during uninterrupted Sandostatin therapy was also observed (Fig. 6): The 24-h plasma GH levels were 12.3 ± 2.8 (mean ± SEM) after 6–12 months of Sandostatin therapy and 5.9 ± 1.6 µg/l after 18–24 months of unchanged medical treatment (p < 0.01). Serum Sm-C concentrations at those time points were 3.7 ± 1.1 and 2.8 ± 0.6 U/ml, respectively (p < 0.01; Fig. 6 right).

In the total group of 10 patients Sm-C and GH levels decreased during Sandostatin therapy by 60% (from 7.3 ± 0.9 to 2.9 ± 0.7 U/ml) and by 87% (from 44.0 ± 7.8 to 5.9 ± 1.0 µg/l), respectively (Fig. 7). Sm-C levels normalized in 5 of these 10 patients. Interestingly, there was a close correlation between the response of circulating GH levels to a first "trial" dose of 50 µg Sandostatin and the degree of suppression of GH levels reached during chronic Sandostatin therapy. There was also a statistically significant correlation between all mean GH levels (the means of the 24-h GH profiles) and Sm-C levels determined before and during therapy in these 10 patients (Fig. 8; n=57; p < 0.001) [17]. This observation

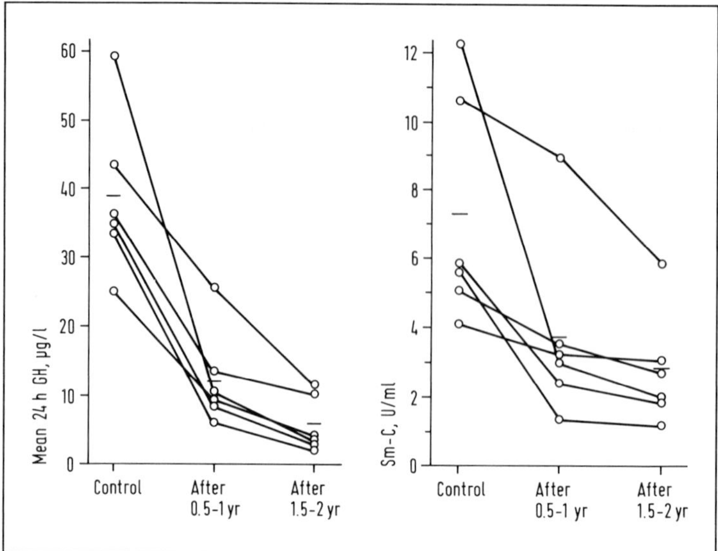

Fig. 6. The course of the mean 24-h growth hormone (GH) levels (left) and somatomedin-C (Sm-C) levels (right) during long-term Sandostatin therapy in 6 acromegalic patients

suggests that an optimal out-patient treatment of acromegalic patients with Sandostatin can be done on the basis of the course of circulating Sm-C levels; there seems no need for extensive measurements of GH profiles.

A slight decrease in pituitary tumor size was observed in about half of the acromegalic patients during Sandostatin therapy [8, 12, 16, 26]. However, tumor size reduc-

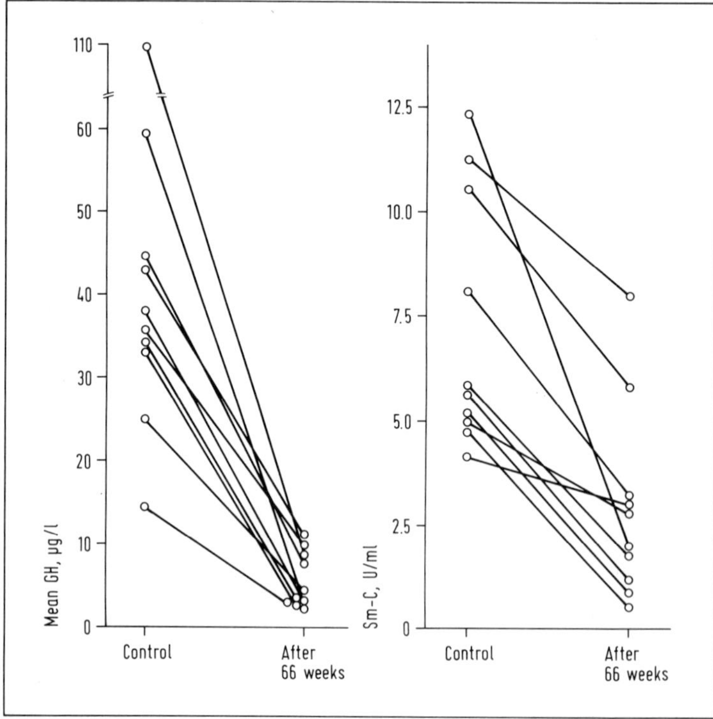

Fig. 7. The effects of chronic treatment of 10 acromegalic patients for a mean of 66 weeks with 200–300 μg Sandostatin per day on mean 24-h growth hormone (GH; left) and somatomedin-C (Sm-C) levels (right)

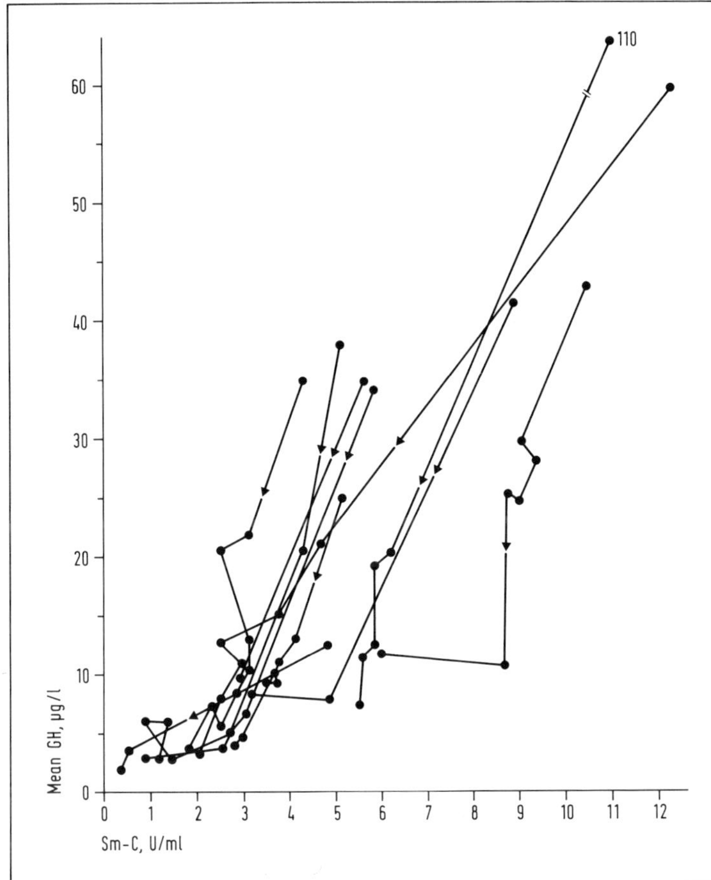

Fig. 8. The course of the mean growth hormone (GH) concentrations (each point is the mean of 20 samples taken over a 24-h period) and the somatomedin-C (Sm-C) concentrations in 10 acromegalics during therapy with 200–300 µg Sandostatin per day for 16–108 weeks (mean 66 weeks). (With kind permission from [17])

tion in these patients, who were treated chronically with, in most instances, 3 × 100 µg Sandostatin per day, was less than that observed during bromocriptine treatment of patients with prolactinomas.

Currently little is known with regard to the mechanism of action of Sandostatin on the GH-secreting pituitary tumors. Four- to five-day administration of Sandostatin to normal rats results in a dose-dependent inhibition of both GH release and GH content of the normal pituitary gland [18]. Culturing GH-secreting pituitary tumor cells in the presence of Sandostatin primarily during the first 24 h inhibits the secretion of GH by the tumor cells, while during longer exposure of the tumor cells to the drug (after 96 h) a decrease of the intracellular GH content of the tumor cells is also observed (Fig. 9) [19]. The shrinkage of these tumors during chronic Sandostatin therapy might well reflect a decrease in the size of the individual tumor cells (caused by the decreased hormone synthesis and hormone content) rather than being the result of a cytotoxic or vascular effect of the drug. In agreement with this assumption are three clinical observations: a) stopping of Sandostatin therapy in acromegaly results in most patients in a rapid increase of circulating GH levels to pretreatment values within days (Fig. 10), while in parallel the symptomatology of acromegaly and pretreatment tumor size are reached within 5–10 days; b) those patients in our series who showed evidence at CT-scanning of slight tumor shrinkage during long-term Sandostatin treatment were those patients in whom the 24-h GH profiles showed a low tendency to increase towards the next injection of the drug. Therefore absence of an increase of serum GH concentrations 5–8 h after the sub-

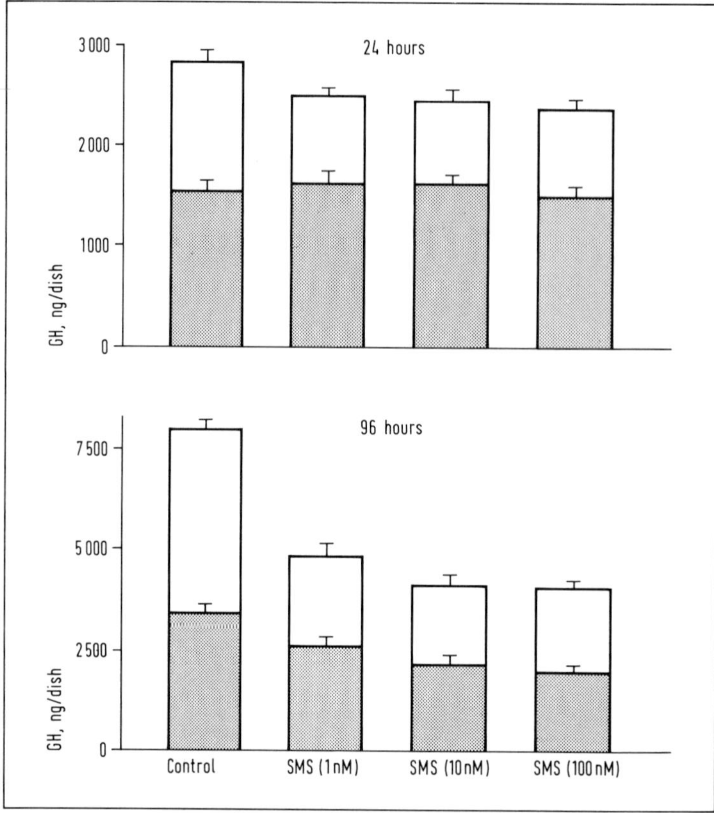

Fig. 9. The effect of Sandostatin on the release and content of growth hormone (GH) in the pituitary tumor cells cultured from a 70-year-old acromegalic female patient. Incubation time 24 h (top) and 96 h (bottom). Open bars represent the amount of GH released into the medium, and hatched bars represent the GH content of the tumor cells (mean ± SEM; n = 4 dishes)

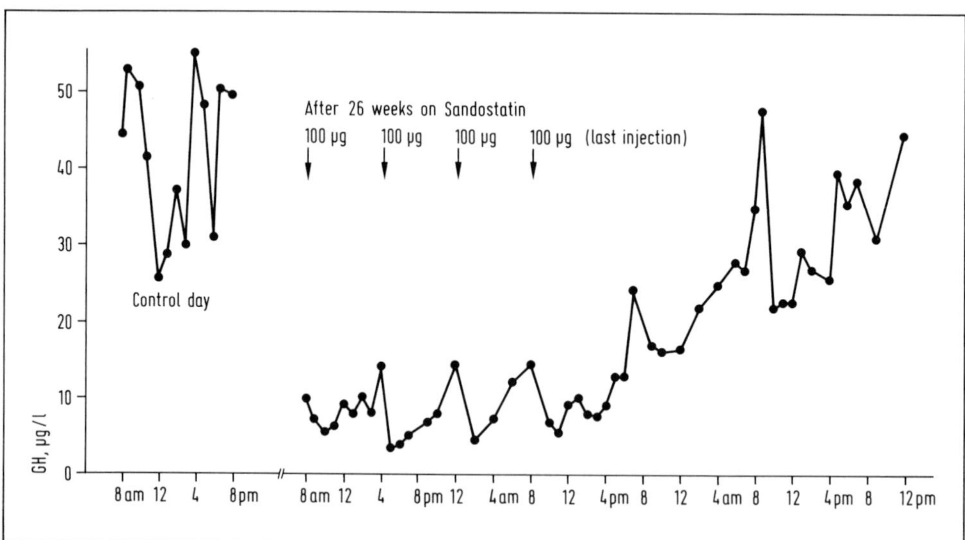

Fig. 10. 24-h growth hormone (GH) profile in an acromegalic patient before and after 26 weeks of Sandostatin (SMS) and for 40 h after the last injection. (With kind permission from [16])

cutaneous injection of Sandostatin during chronic therapy might not only reflect a high sensitivity of this tumor to the drug (high number of and/or high affinity of the somatostatin receptors), but also a decrease in the intratumoral GH synthesis and content. c) Ducasse et al. [6] observed much more impressive tumor shrinkage in their acromegalic patient during chronic therapy with Sandostatin, but these investigators administered the drug with a constant 24-h infusion during many months. This therapeutic approach suppressed GH levels over the complete period of drug administration and this presumably might result in a more profound emptying of the GH-secreting tumor cells.

Comparison of the Effects of Sandostatin and Bromocriptine

We compared the acute GH-inhibitory effects of 50 µg Sandostatin and of 2.5 mg bromocriptine in 17 acromegalic patients [14]. Sandostatin suppressed plasma GH concentrations after 2−6 h to 5 µg/l or less in 10 of these 17 patients, while bromocriptine produced similar results in only 5 of them. There was no homogeneity in the responsiveness to either drug in the patients studied, but the GH-lowering effect of 50 µg Sandostatin was significantly greater than that elicited by 2.5 mg bromocriptine (Fig. 11). In all patients together the effect of the combination of both drugs did not cause a more profound suppression of GH levels than Sandostatin alone. Sandostatin and bromocriptine together significantly suppressed plasma GH levels in 2 of 3 acro-

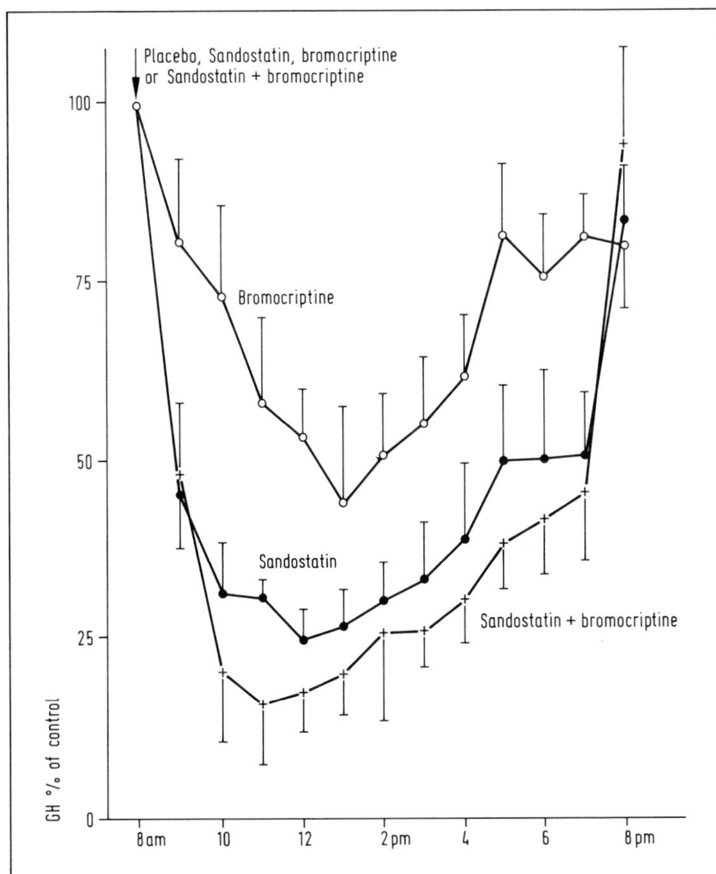

Fig. 11. Mean (± SEM) percent change in plasma growth hormone (GH) levels after Sandostatin, bromocriptine and the combination of both compounds compared with values after placebo injection in 7 acromegalic patients. (With kind permission from [14])

megalic patients who were insensitive to both compounds tested separately. Most acromegalic patients in this study responded better to Sandostatin, while a few patients were more sensitive to the GH-lowering effect of bromocriptine. The combination of both Sandostatin and bromocriptine can probably be of value in a few acromegalic patients who do not respond to either of these drugs separately [14].

The Effect of Sandostatin on Prolactin Secretion

We reported before that the sensitivity of GH secretion to bromocriptine in acromegaly increases significantly in the GH-secreting pituitary adenomas which simultaneously synthesize PRL [13]. We therefore also investigated whether immunohistologically detectable PRL in a GH-secreting pituitary tumor and/or the level of the plasma PRL concentration might play a role in determining the sensitivity of GH as well as of PRL secretion to Sandostatin [15]. In a group of 18 patients with acromegaly we

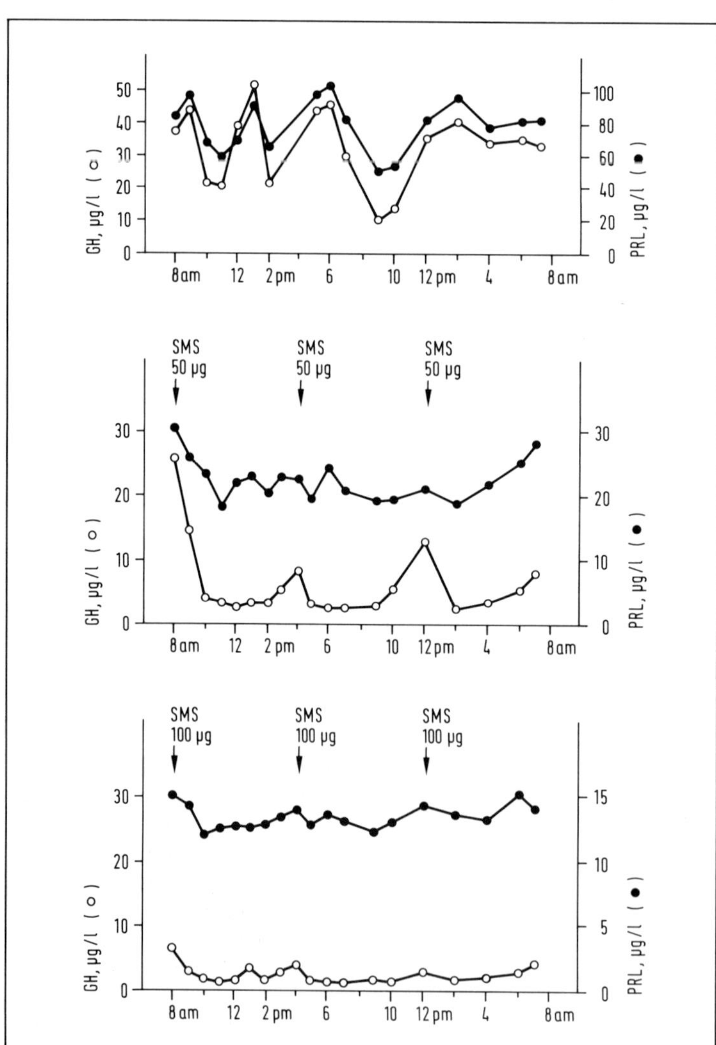

Fig. 12. The effect of long-term therapy with Sandostatin (SMS) on circulating growth hormone (GH) and prolactin (PRL) levels in a patient with a mixed GH/PRL-containing pituitary tumor. *Top panel*: control day. *Middle panel*: after 3 weeks of therapy with 3 × 50 µg Sandostatin subcutaneously. *Lower panel*: after 16 weeks of therapy with 3 × 100 µg Sandostatin. (O) GH, (●) PRL levels. (With kind permission from [14])

found 11 pure GH-secreting tumors, while mixed GH/PRL-containing adenomas were found in the other 7 patients. In two of these "mixed" tumors there was evidence for GH and PRL being secreted by the same tumor cells. The sensitivity of GH secretion to Sandostatin was not different in the patients with pure GH- or mixed GH/PRL-containing adenomas. Plasma PRL levels were not affected by Sandostatin in the patients with pure GH-secreting tumors, but were significantly suppressed in 4 of the 7 patients with mixed GH/PRL-containing tumors. One of these patients was treated for 16 weeks with 300 µg Sandostatin daily. The mean GH levels decreased from 34.2 ± 3.0 µg/l (Fig. 12, top) to 2.6 ± 0.3 µg/l (Fig. 12, bottom), respectively (mean of 20 samples ± SEM), while plasma PRL levels also normalized from 79.4 ± 4.0 µg/l to 13.6 ± 0.2 µg/l during therapy. In contrast, hyperprolactinemia in four patients with microprolactinomas was not suppressed by Sandostatin [15]. Interestingly, we also have preliminary evidence that the elevated circulating α-subunit concentrations which can be found in about 20% of acromegalic patients respond to Sandostatin in close parallel to the changes in GH secretion.

Side Effects

All acromegalic patients studied responded well both to the acute administration as well as to self-administration of Sandostatin. The injection sites on the anterior aspect of each thigh remained soft. Transient abdominal discomfort occurred in 2 out of 10 patients during the first week of chronic therapy, while transient steatorrhea was observed in 2 other patients.

Mean fasting serum glucose concentrations did not change during chronic treatment with 200–300 µg Sandostatin per day in eight of ten patients who had normal carbohydrate tolerance before therapy. Figure 13 shows the glucose and insulin concentrations before and after breakfast and dinner on a control day, after a single dose of 50 µg Sandostatin and after the administration of 100 µg Sandostatin, three times daily, at the end of the long-term treatment period in these eight patients. Sandostatin was given 30 min before breakfast and 2 h before dinner. It is evident that moderate hyperglycemia followed breakfast both after a single dose and during long-term therapy. This increase in glucose levels coincided with transient inhibition of insulin secretion. The area under the curve of glucose concentrations from 90–100 min after breakfast remained significantly increased both after a single dose and during long-term therapy (p < 0.01 and p < 0.05, respectively). Thus, there was no evidence for the development of tolerance or tachyphylaxis of the inhibitory effect on insulin release during long-term therapy.

Two of these 10 patients had type 2 diabetes mellitus initially. In one of them the sulfonylureas used at first could be stopped during Sandostatin therapy, while in the other the initially marginally increased glucose levels further increased. Treatment with a sulfonylurea derivative, however, overcame the inhibitory effect of Sandostatin on insulin release and normalized fasting and postprandial glucose concentrations.

Conclusions

The clinical introduction of the long-acting somatostatin analog Sandostatin adds a new dimension to the therapy of acromegaly which cannot be cured by surgery and/or radiotherapy. Sandostatin is in most patients much more effective than bromocriptine. In all patients a marked clinical improvement can be expected in the first weeks of therapy with the drug while hardly any side effects occur. Sandostatin in a dose of 300 µg/day in three subcutaneous injections eventually normalized Sm-C levels in about 50% of patients. Interestingly, a gradual continuous decline in Sm-C levels was observed during therapy for over one year with Sandostatin. A slight decrease in tumor size occurs in about half of the patients treated with 300 µg Sandostatin. A possible mechanism of action is shrinkage of the size of individual tumor cells which cease to synthesize GH and which contain less GH. Preliminary evidence suggests that continuous intravenous administration of Sandostatin will eventually result in a more

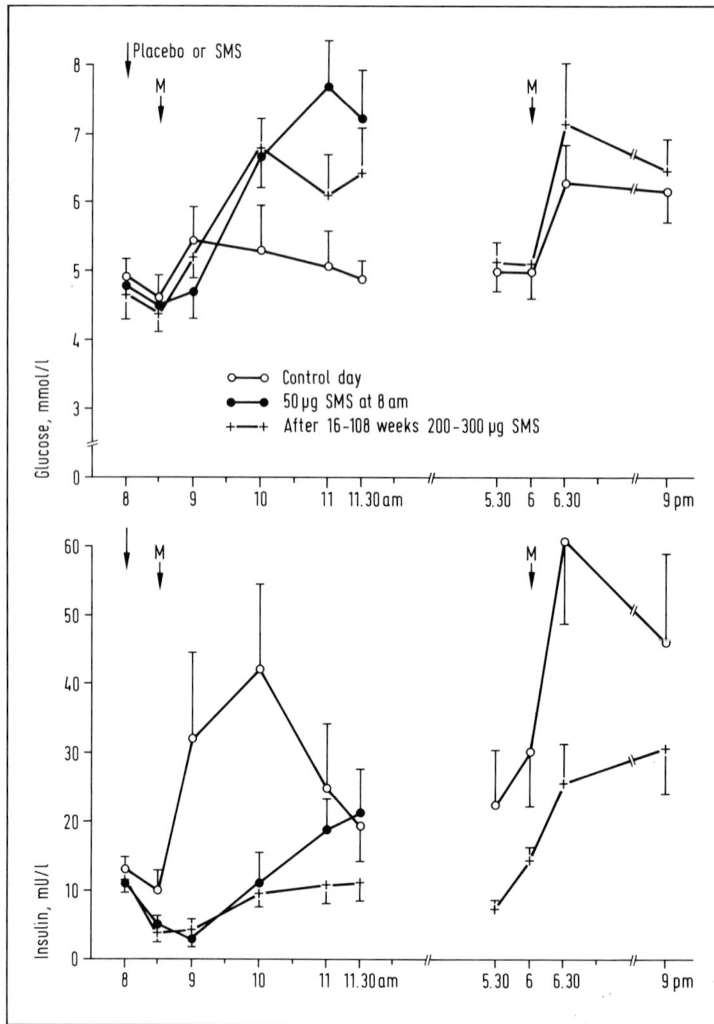

Fig. 13. Mean (± SEM) serum glucose and insulin profiles before and during Sandostatin therapy in 8 acromegalic patients during a control day, after the first dose of 50 µg Sandostatin (SMS), and at the end of long-term treatment with daily doses of 200−300 µg Sandostatin. M = meal. (With kind permission from [16])

impressive tumor shrinkage than intermittent subcutaneous administration. However, the effects of Sandostatin in acromegaly are reversible and both pretreatment GH/Sm-C levels and tumor size reappear within days to weeks after stopping chronic Sandostatin therapy.

Sandostatin represents a new, exciting addition to the medical management of acromegaly. At present we treat those patients with Sandostatin who did not benefit from surgical therapy, or in whom the effects of radiotherapy have to be awaited. In addition, however, we also currently start Sandostatin therapy in otherwise untreated patients in whom a surgical procedure is considered to be hazardous. The low toxicity of the drug might make it eventually the first treatment of choice in most acromegalics.

References

1. Barnard LB, Granthan WG, Lamberton P, O'Dorisio TM, Jackson IMD (1986) Treatment of resistant acromegaly with a long-acting somatostatin analogue (SMS 201-995). Ann Intern Med 105:856−862
2. Bauer W, Briner U, Doepfner W, Haller R, Huguenin R, Marbach P, Petcher TJ, Pless J (1982) SMS 201-995: a very potent and selective octapeptide analogue of somatostatin

with prolonged action. Life Sci 31: 1133−1141

3. Brazeau P, Vale W, Burgus R, Ling N, Butcher M, Rivier J, Guillemin R (1973) Hypothalamic polypeptide that inhibits the secretion of immunoreactive pituitary growth hormone. Science 179:77−79

4. Chiodini PG, Cozzi R, Dallabonzana D, Oppizzi G, Verde G, Petroncini M, Liuzzi A, Del Pozo E (1987) Medical treatment of acromegaly with SMS 201-995, a somatostatin analog: A comparison with bromocriptine. J Clin Endocrinol Metab 64: 447−453

5. Ch'ng IJC, Sandler IM, Kraenzlin ME, Burrin JM, Joplin GF, Bloom SR (1985) Long-term treatment of acromegaly with a long-acting analogue of somatostatin. Br Med J 290:284−285

6. Ducasse MCR, Tauber JP, Tourre A (1987) Dramatic shrinking effect of somatostatin analogue SMS 201-995 on GH-producing pituitary tumours. J Clin Endocrinol Metab (in press)

7. Del Pozo E, Neufeld M, Schlütter K, Tortosa F, Clarenbach P, Bieder E, Wendel I, Nüesch E, Marbach P, Cramer H, Kerp I (1986) Endocrine profile of a long-acting somatostatin derivative SMS 201-995. Study in normal volunteers following subcutaneous administration. Acta Endocrinol 111: 433−439

8. Jackson I, Barnard LB, Lamberton P (1986) Role of a long-acting somatostatin analogue (SMS 201-995) in the treatment of acromegaly. Am J Med 81(6b):94−99

9. Lamberts SWJ, Del Pozo E (1986) Acute and long-term effects of SMS 201-995 in acromegaly. Scand J Gastroenterol 21(119): 141−149

10. Lamberts SWJ, Verleun T, Oosterom R (1984) The interrelationship between the effects of somatostatin and human pancreatic growth hormone releasing factor on growth hormone release by cultured pituitary tumor cells from patients with acromegaly. J Clin Endocrinol Metab 58:250−255

11. Lamberts SWJ, Oosterom R, Neufeld M, Del Pozo E (1985) The somatostatin analog SMS 201-995 induces long-acting inhibition of growth hormone secretion without rebound hypersecretion in acromegalic patients. J Clin Endocrinol Metab 60: 1161−1165

12. Lamberts SWJ, Uitterlinden P, Verschoor L, van Dongen KJ, Del Pozo E (1985) Long-term treatment of acromegaly with the somatostatin analogue SMS 201-995. N Engl J Med 313:1576−1580

13. Lamberts SWJ, Klijn JGM, van Vroonhoven CCJ, Stefanko SZ (1985) Different responses of growth hormone secretion to guanfacine, bromocriptine, and thyrotropin-releasing hormone in acromegalic patients with pure growth hormone (GH)-containing and mixed GH/proclactin-containing pituitary adenomas. J Clin Endocrinol Metab 60: 1148−1153

14. Lamberts SWJ, Zweens M, Verschoor L, Del Pozo E (1986) A comparison among the growth hormone-lowering effects in acromegaly of the somatostatin analog SMS 201-995, bromocriptine, and the combination of both drugs. J Clin Endocrinol Metab 63:16−19

15. Lamberts SWJ, Zweens M, Klijn JGM, van Vroonhoven CCJ, Stefanko SZ, Del Pozo E (1986) The sensitivity of growth hormone and prolactin secretion to the somatostatin analogue SMS 201-995 in patients with prolactinomas and acromegaly. Clin Endocrinol 25:201−212

16. Lamberts SWJ, Uitterlinden P, Del Pozo E (1987) Sandostatin (SMS 201-995) induces a continuous further decline in circulating growth hormone and somatomedin-C levels during therapy of acromegalic patients for over two years. J Clin Endocrinol Metab 65:703−710

17. Lamberts SWJ, Uitterlinden P, Verleun T (1987) The relationship between growth hormone and somatomedin-C levels in untreated acromegaly, after surgery and radiotherapy and during medical therapy with Sandostatin (SMS 201-995). Eur J Clin Invest 17:354−359

18. Lamberts SWJ, Verleun T, Zuiderwijk JM, Oosterom R (1987) The effect of the somatostatin analog SMS 201-995 on normal growth hormone secretion in the rat. A comparison with the effect of bromocriptine on normal prolactin secretion. Acta Endocrinol 115:196−202

19. Lamberts SWJ, Verleun T, Hofland LJ, Del Pozo E (1987) A comparison between the effects of Sandostatin (SMS 201-995), bromocriptine and a combination of both drugs on hormone release by the cultured pituitary tumour cells of acromegalic patients. Clin Endocrinol 27:11−23

20. Oppizzi G, Petroncini MM, Dallabonzana D, Cozzi R, Verde G, Chiodini PG, Liuzzi A (1986) Relationship between somatomedin-C and growth hormone levels in acromegaly: basal and dynamic evaluation. J Clin Endocrinol Metab 63:1348−1353

21. Pieters GFFM, van Liessum PA, Smals AGH, van Gennep JA, Benraad ThJ, Kloppenborg PWC (1987) Long-term treatment of acromegaly with Sandostatin (SMS 201-995), normalization of most anomalous

growth hormone responses. Acta Endocrinol (in press)

22. Plewe G, Beyer J, Krause U, Neufeld M, Del Pozo E (1984) Long-acting and selective suppression of growth hormone secretion by somatostatin analogue SMS 201-995 in acromegaly. Lancet II:782−784

23. Plewe G, Schrezenmeir J, Nölken G, Krause U, Beyer J, Kasper H, Del Pozo E (1986) Long-term treatment of acromegaly with the somatostatin analogue SMS 201-995 over 6 months. Klin Wochenschr 64:389−392

24. Reubi JC, Landolt AM (1984) High density of somatostatin receptors in pituitary tumors from acromegalic patients. J Clin Endocrinol 59: 1148−1153

25. Williams G, Burrin JM, Ball JA, Joplin GF, Bloom SR (1986) Effective and lasting growth-hormone suppression in active acromegaly with oral administration of somatostatin analogue SMS 201-995. Lancet II: 774−777

26. Wilson DM, Hoffman AR (1986) Reduction of pituitary size by the somatostatin analogue SMS 201-995 in a patient with an islet cell tumour secreting growth hormone releasing factor. Acta Endocrinol 113:23−28

9. Medical Treatment of Acromegaly. Dopaminergic Agonists and Long-Acting Somatostatin

A. Liuzzi, P. G. Chiodini, R. Cozzi, D. Dallabonzana, G. Oppizzi, M. M. Petroncini

Divisione di Endocrinologia, Ospedale Niguarda, Milano, Italy

The medical treatment of acromegaly is of value because neurosurgery and Rx therapy may be unsuccessful in this disease.

The goal of a stable pharmacological suppression of GH levels in acromegaly was achieved [3] by the use of the long-lasting dopaminergic drug bromocriptine (Br). However, less than 30% of the patients have their GH and somatomedin-C (Sm-C) levels normalized and multiple daily administrations of Br are required.

Recently, a somatostatin analog with long-lasting inhibitory activity on GH release (SMS 201-995, Sandostatin®) has been made available for clinical use. The data so far collected indicate that this agent improves the effectiveness of the pharmacological treatment of this disease.

The aim of this work is to summarize our own experience on the use of Sandostatin in the medical treatment of acromegaly.

There is already evidence [4, 5, 7, 8, 10] that Sandostatin reduces GH levels in acromegalic patients and reverses the metabolic consequences of the hypersecretion of this hormone. The effect of the drug is already evident on the first day of treatment and persists even for prolonged periods of up to two years.

We have studied the effects of Sandostatin given either by multiple subcutaneous injections or by continuous subcutaneous infusion with a minipump, on a large series of acromegalic patients during long-term treatment with Sandostatin.

Multiple Daily Injections

We have treated 26 patients with Sandostatin given by multiple subcutaneous injections at doses of $100-1500$ µg daily for $3-27$ months. These dosages, divided into $2-3$ subcutaneous injections, reduced GH and Sm-C levels in the majority of the patients studied but with a wide intersubject variability (Fig. 1). Basal plasma GH (55.8 ± 8 ng/ml) and Sm-C levels (8.6 ± 4 U/ml) significantly decreased by the second day, and fell after 15 days of treatment to 12 ± 3 ng/ml ($p < 0.01$) and to 2.5 ± 0.6 U/ml ($p < 0.05$) respectively. Thereafter there were no further significant changes in GH and Sm-C levels even in the patients treated for up to 27 months. The mean daily GH profile showed a maximum GH inhibition within $2-3$ h after Sandostatin administration and a progressive return close to preinjection values within $6-12$ h. This GH pattern was, however, less evident when 100 µg or more t.i.d. were used. Moreover, GH levels were in the normal range throughout the day in only 4 of 9 patients treated with these dosages. Collectively, 22 of the 26 patients (85%) had their GH and Sm-C levels reduced by SMS. In a few patients a true refractoriness to the drug activity could be demonstrated; in particular, one patient failed to reduce her GH levels even when given 1500 µg/day of the drug.

Comparison of Br and Sandostatin

A comparison between the long-term effects of Br (20 mg/day) and Sandostatin ($100-300$ µg/day) performed in 13 out of these 26 patients, revealed that SMS induced a greater GH and Sm-C inhibition than Br. Plasma GH and Sm-C levels were lower during Sandostatin than Br in 11 of the 13 patients; in addition only 13% of the patients were unresponsive to Sandostatin whereas 50% of them did not respond to Br.

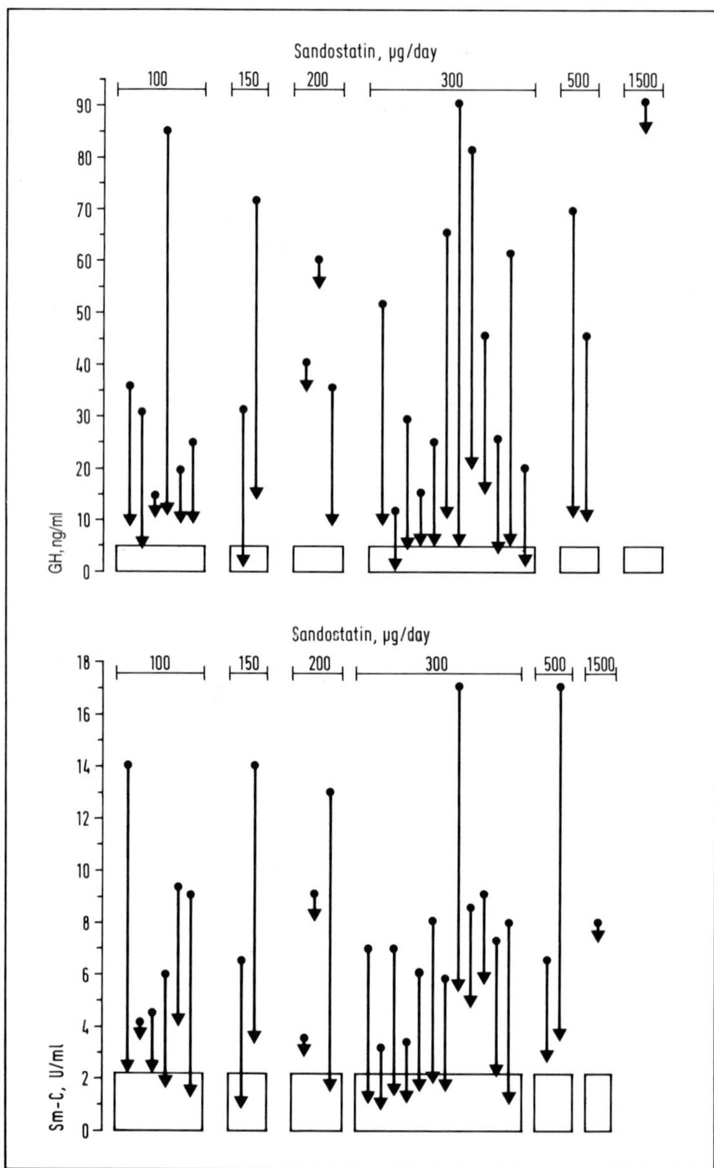

Fig. 1. Mean growth hormone (GH) (ng/ml) and somatomedin-C (Sm-C) (U/ml) levels during treatment with Sandostatin in 26 acromegalic patients

Continuous Infusion of Sandostatin

The effects of Sandostatin given at dosages ranging from 50 µg b.i.d. to 200 µg t.i.d. either by multiple subcutaneous injections or by continuous infusion were studied. Equivalent doses of the drug were given to each patient by multiple subcutaneous injections and subsequently by continuous infusion, or vice versa, for at least two months; the two treatments were separated by a washout period of one month.

GH and Sm-C levels fell significantly with either kind of treatment within the second day but, during continuous infusion, a significantly more marked decrease of GH and Sm-C was observed.

The analytical evaluation of the data showed that plasma GH and Sm-C levels were reduced but not normalized during

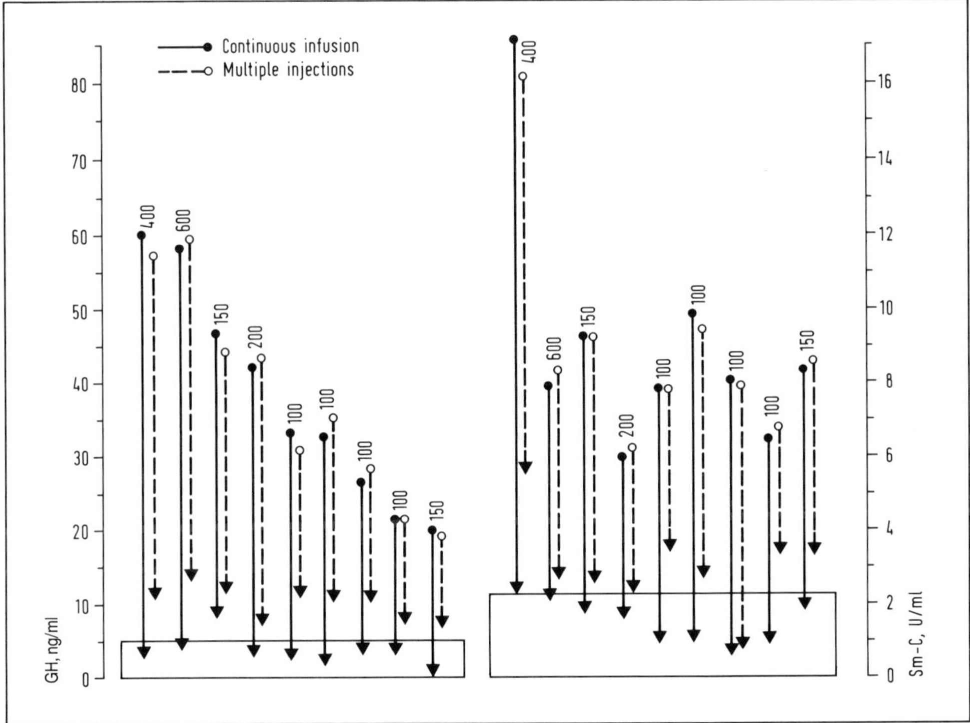

Fig. 2. Growth hormone (GH) and somatomedin-C (Sm-C) levels during treatment with Sandostatin given to the same patient either by multiple subcutaneous injections or by continuous infusion. The numbers over the arrows indicate the daily dosage of Sandostatin (µg/day)

multiple subcutaneous injections, whereas they fell into the normal range in all patients during continuous infusion (Fig. 2).

The prolongation of continuous infusion treatment for 12–18 months in 4 patients showed GH and Sm-C levels to be stable within the normal range but the withdrawal of the therapy was followed by the return of GH and Sm-C to pretreatment levels within 24–36 h.

Effects of Sandostatin Treatment on the Clinical and Metabolic Parameters

The decrease of the GH levels was accompanied by an amelioration of the signs and symptoms of the disease as well as of the metabolic alterations related to GH hypersecretion. Serum procollagen III propeptide (i.e. PIIIP) levels fell (p < 0.01) from 16.5 ± 1.8 to 8.4 ± 0.5 ng/ml. Overt diabetes improved in two of the three diabetics and in

one of them insulin therapy could be stopped. Slight postprandial hyperglycemia occurred in 6 patients whose glucose tolerance was previously normal. Fasting and postprandial serum insulin did not significantly change during treatment.

CT scan showed, in comparable coronal sections, a reduction in tumor size in 10 out of the 20 patients with evidence of a large adenoma. This number of tumor size reductions, observed also by others [1, 7, 8, 11] is greater than that observed during Br treatment, and suggests that Sandostatin also exerts an antitumoral effect on GH-secreting adenomas.

Conclusions

The chronic treatment with Sandostatin induced a long-term GH and Sm-C suppression in 85% of our patients, in accordance with the results reported by other authors

[2, 7–10]. During treatment prolonged up to 27 months, the degree of GH suppression, in relation to the dosage employed, was unchanged; this finding indicates that desensitization of the pituitary receptors to somatostatin does not occur during Sandostatin treatment. The results of the dose-response study show that a satisfactory control of GH hypersecretion during Sandostatin by multiple subcutaneous injections is dependent on both the timing of administration and the dose, since a stable normalization of GH levels was only obtained with 300 µg t.i.d.

A stable GH suppression to normal levels throughout the day may not, however, be necessary to control the disease, since plasma Sm-C fell into the normal range in 7 patients whose GH levels were not normal over a 24-h period. In addition, an impressive improvement in clinical symptoms and of metabolic alterations due to GH hypersecretion was observed in most patients during the treatment, even when plasma GH and Sm-C were not normalized.

We did not find any consistent long-term changes in glucose tolerance in the patients with previously normal blood glucose in agreement with the data of Lamberts et al. [7], and insulin levels were not suppressed by Sandostatin treatment as might have been expected. On the contrary, diabetes improved, probably as a consequence of the GH suppression induced by Sandostatin.

The comparative evaluation of the results obtained with Sandostatin and Br is of clinical and pathophysiological interest: 100–300 µg/day of Sandostatin was actually more effective in reducing GH and Sm-C levels than 20 mg/day of Br. Since, in our experience, higher Br dosages do not achieve any further suppression of GH levels, we may conclude that the chronic GH lowering effect of Sandostatin is more pronounced than that of Br. In previous studies [1, 7, 8, 11] a slight reduction of tumor size was observed during chronic Sandostatin administration.

In the present series the tumor shrank in 10 out 20 patients so far examined by CT. These findings indicate that Sandostatin may exert an antitumoral effect on the GH-secreting adenomas. In vitro studies [6] performed on adenomas from patients oper-

ated on after Sandostatin treatment have shown only a reduction of cellular volume; this is in agreement with the clinical finding that GH levels revert to the pretreatment values soon after drug withdrawal.

In conclusion, Sandostatin is a more effective agent than Br in the medical treatment of acromegaly and may be considered, especially when given by continuous infusion, the drug of first choice. In fact the percentage of patients whose GH and Sm-C are normalized, or at least markedly reduced, is far higher than that clearly established for the dopamine agonists. In addition, in our experience tumor shrinkage is more frequent with Sandostatin than with the long-acting dopaminergic compounds which, however, can represent, for selected patients, an effective and more practical alternative to Sandostatin treatment.

(This study was supported by the National Research Council, special project Oncology, Grant No. 86.00675.44)

References

1. Barnard L (1986) Reduction of pituitary tumor size in acromegaly treated with a somatostatin analogue (SMS 201-995). 68th Meeting of Endocrine Society, June 25–27, Anaheim, abstract 983
2. Ch'ng LJC, Sandler LM, Kraenzli ME, Burrin JM, Joplin JF, Bloom SR (1985) Long term treatment of acromegaly with a long acting analog. Br Med J 290:284–287
3. Chiodini PG, Liuzzi A, Botalla L, Oppizzi G, Muller EE, Silvestrini F (1975) Stable reduction of plasma growth hormone (hGH) levels during chronic administration of 2Br-alfa-ergocryptine (CB 154) in acromegalic patients. J Clin Endocrinol Metab 40: 705–708
4. Chiodini PG, Cozzi R, Dallabonzana D, Oppizzi G, Verde G, Petroncini M, Liuzzi A, Del Pozo E (1987) Medical treatment of acromegaly with SMS 201-995, a somatostatin analog: a comparison with bromocriptine. J Clin Endocrinol Metab 64:447–450
5. Cozzi R, Chiodini PG, Dallabonzana D, Petroncini M, Verde G, Oppizzi G, Liuzzi A (1986) Effect of SMS 201-995 administered by minipump infusion in acromegaly. International Conference on somatostatin, Washington, May 6–8, 1987, p 64
6. George SR, Kovacs K, Asa SL, Horvath E,

Cross EG, Burrow GN (1987) Effect of SMS 201-995, a long-acting somatostatin analogue, on the secretion and morphology of a pituitary growth hormone cell adenoma. Clin Endocrinol (Oxf) 26:395

7. Lamberts SWJ, Uitterlinden P, Verschoor L, van Dongen KJ, Del Pozo E (1985) Long term treatment of acromegaly with the somatostatin analogue SMS 201-995. N Engl J Med 313:1576–1578

8. Lamberts SWJ, Uitterlinden P, Del Pozo E (1987) SMS 201-995 induces a continuous decline in circulating growth hormone and somatomedin-C levels during therapy of acromegalic patients for over two years. J Clin Endocrinol Metab 65:704

9. Landolt AM, Osterwalder V, Jantzer R, Stuckmann G (1985) The medical treatment of acromegaly with lisuride. Neuroendocrinol Lett 2:94–96

10. Plewe G, Beyer J, Krause U, Neufeld M, Del Pozo E (1984) Long acting and selective suppression of growth hormone secretion by somatostatin analogue SMS 201-995 in acromegaly. Lancet II:782–784

11. Tolis G, Yotis A, Malachtari S, Rigas G, Hortoglou A, Del Pozo E, Andreu I, Papavasileiu C (1986) Follow-up of acromegalic patients treated with an octapeptide somatostatin analogue for over a year. 68th Meeting of Endocrine Society, June 25– Anaheim, abstract 746

10. Treatment of Acromegaly with the Somatostatin Analogue SMS 201-995 (Sandostatin®)

H.-J. Quabbe, U. Plöckinger

Department of Internal Medicine, Section of Endocrinology, Klinikum Steglitz, Freie Universität, Berlin, FRG

The long-acting somatostatin analogue SMS 201-995 (Sandostatin®) has recently been introduced for the treatment of acromegaly [1]. We have evaluated its efficacy and long-term usefulness in 12 patients with therapy-resistant disease. All had been previously treated by transsphenoidal surgery, irradiation, bromocriptine or a combination of these but their GH concentrations had been insufficiently lowered. Duration of Sandostatin treatment was at least 12 months in all patients.

Methods

Sandostatin was injected subcutaneously at doses of 3×100, 3×200 and 3×500 µg/d respectively. Hourly blood samples were obtained for 24-h periods for the determination of growth hormone (GH), prolactin (PRL), insulin and blood glucose (BG). Somatomedin-C (Sm-C[1]) was determined in the first three samples of each profile. Profiles were obtained before therapy and after 2 weeks on each dose. In addition, GH, insulin and BG were also determined during oral glucose loading (100 g, OGTT) which was done on the day after each profile. Following evaluation of GH and somatomedin-C results obtained during the increasing Sandostatin doses, patients were kept on an individually adjusted dose of Sandostatin, which had provided maximal GH and/or Sm-C suppression. Comparison of the three time periods following each s.c. injection of Sandostatin showed that the

GH concentrations were not significantly different between these time periods. Therefore, it was possible to compare 8-h periods (08.00−16.00) of the 24-h profiles with an 8-h profile done after one year of treatment. Wilcoxon's signed ranks test for paired samples was used for statistical evaluation of differences between treatment periods. The study was explained in detail to each patient and his/her written consent was obtained. It was approved by the hospital ethical committee.

Results

During Sandostatin therapy the mean 24-h GH concentration was reduced in 8/12 patients to $11-55\%$ of their baseline concentration. In the other 4 patients the GH concentration during therapy was not significantly lower on the highest dose (3×500 µg/d) than during baseline conditions. Mean GH ($\pm$ SE) in the total group decreased from 14.5 ± 5.8 to 4.9 ± 1.8, 5.0 ± 2.2, 4.3 ± 1.8 and 4.9 ± 1.7 ng/ml on 3×100, 3×200, 3×500 µg/d and the individual dose respectively. The mean GH suppression during the various Sandostatin doses was not significantly different. However, when the 8 responders were analysed individually, four of them had significantly lower GH concentrations on 3×200 µg/d or 3×500 µg/d than on the lower doses. When the GH and Sm-C concentrations of all treatment doses were available, one patient was omitted from further treatment because of non-response. One patient discontinued treatment despite significant lowering of her GH concentration.

Sm-C decreased in 11/12 patients. The mean Sm-C concentration ($\pm$ SE) de-

---

[1] Sm-C was kindly determined through the courtesy of Dr. A. G. Harris, Sandoz Ltd, Basle, Switzerland

creased from 2.5 ± 0.1 to 1.5 ± 0.0, 1.0 ± 0.1, 1.1 ± 0.0 U/ml on 3 × 100, 3 × 200 and 3 × 500 µg/d, respectively. In several patients a dissociation between the responses of GH and Sm-C to Sandostatin treatment was observed. In one patient (a GH non-responder) the 24-h mean GH was relatively low (4.0 ng/ml) but her Sm-C concentration was high (> 4 U/ml) irrespective of the Sandostatin dose (GH and Sm-C non-responder). In 4 other patients − including the 3 other GH non-responders − the Sm-C decrease was more pronounced than the GH decrease. Therefore, in these three patients treatment was continued despite the absence of a GH response.

After one year of treatment, mean GH concentration in the remaining 10 patients was 4.1 ± 1.3 ng/ml when tested in an 8-h profile and hence was slightly lower than during treatment with 3 × 500 µg/d although 7 of the 10 patients had been on long-term treatment with only 3 × 100 µg/d.

The PRL concentration was within normal limits in all patients before treatment. It decreased slightly but significantly during the dose-response study (from 11.9 ± 2.5 to 9.3 ± 1.8, 9.1 ± 1.8 and 8.9 ± 1.8 µg/l respectively).

Two patients had manifest diabetes mellitus when entering the study. Their values were omitted from the analysis of the insulin and BG concentrations. The mean 24-h insulin concentration decreased from 23.7 ± 2.8 to 14.1 ± 1.3, 11.4 ± 0.7 and 11.7 ± 1.7 mIU/l during the different treatment doses. BG increased to 128% of the pretreatment concentration on 3 × 100 µg Sandostatin but then declined again despite the continuation of treatment. None of the patients developed manifest diabetes mellitus during treatment.

During oral glucose loading GH was not suppressed below 1 ng/ml in any patient before treatment with Sandostatin. It became suppressible below this concentration (lower limit of the sensitivity of the GH radioimmunoassay) in 4/10 patients during Sandostatin treatment.

Side effects consisted mostly of loose stools and flatulence but decreased with continuing therapy in spite of dose increases. No patient discontinued treatment because of side effects.

Conclusions

Sandostatin effectively suppressed GH concentrations in 8/12 patients with previously therapy-resistant acromegaly while Sm-C concentrations were lowered in 11 of these 12 patients. In four patients a dose of 100 µg of Sandostatin given three times per day provided maximal GH suppression. In the other four patients a higher dose was slightly more effective. Glucose tolerance decreased in the presence of suppressed insulin concentrations but manifest diabetes mellitus did not develop. During a 1-year period, escape from the treatment effect did not occur.

Reference

1. Bauer W, Briner U, Doepfner W, Haller R, Huguenin R, Marbach P, Petcher TJ, Pless J (1982) SMS 201-995: A very potent and selective octapeptide analogue of somatostatin with prolonged action. Life Sci 31:1133−1140

11. Observations During a Clinical Trial of Sandostatin® in Acromegalic Patients

H. Ørskov[1], J. Weeke[2], S. E. Christensen[2], S. Nielsen[1], A. Flyvbjerg[2], J. O. L. Jørgensen[2], N. Møller[1], A. G. Harris[3]

[1] Institute of Experimental Clinical Research, University of Aarhus, Denmark, [2] Second University Clinic of Internal Medicine, Kommunehospitalet, Aarhus, Denmark, [3] Pharma Division, Clinical Research, Sandoz Ltd, Basle, Switzerland

Patients, Serum GH and Sandostatin® Administration Protocol

Ten acromegalic patients were studied over a period of 75 weeks. Four had had one or more attempted ablations of their pituitary adenoma, six were previously untreated or had been unsuccessfully treated with bromocriptine. At entrance to the study they had 24-h serum growth hormone means ranging from 19.4 to 154 ng/ml and pronounced clinical evidence of active acromegaly.

During the study each patient was admitted to the hospital on 28 occasions and underwent 12- or 24-h profiles of serum GH, insulin, glucose, TSH, T3, T4, Sandostatin and somatomedin-C levels as well as clinical evaluation and safety parameters. No side effects were noted apart from transient slight abdominal discomfort and loose stools just after increase of Sandostatin doses.

Figures 1 and 2 show the serum growth hormone (GH) patterns in two patients between 8 am and noon (which we find illustrates the efficacy of the Sandostatin treatment, as it includes the frequently high morning serum GH level) during the entire study and during the increases in Sandostatin dosage indicated on the abscissa.

During the initial part (7 days) of the study, pretreatment GH levels were compared with those observed after 3 days' administration of 100 μg/24 h Sandostatin given subcutaneously by constant pump infusion and with those observed after another 3 days, when the same amount was injected as 3 equally spaced subcutaneous injections of 33 + 33 + 33 μg/24 h. The results have been described previously in detail [1]. In brief, better and more constant suppression was attained during pump treatment. One day after withdrawal, pretreatment serum GH levels were re-attained.

After about one month Sandostatin administration was resumed comparing one month's continuous subcutaneous infusion (CSI) of 250 μg/24 h with a period during which the diurnal dose was divided into injections of 50 + 50 + 50 + 100 μg. The trial continued according to the Sandostatin Multicenter Study protocol ending up with 500 μg given 3 times/24 h. Finally, this schedule was compared with the effect of CSI of 1500 μg/24 h.

Generally, better and more constant serum GH suppression was attained with CSI infusions than with the same dose administered as 3 or 4 daily injections. In most patients a daily dose of 600 μg was more effective than lower or higher ones.

Six patients achieved suppression of average 24-h serum GH levels to below 5 ng/ml, while the other 4 had clearly insufficient inhibition of 24-h GH release to minimum 24-h serum levels of 17.5; 39.0; 43.4 and 60.6 ng/ml.

We should like to discuss two of the observations we found of interest during the trial.

Carbohydrate Tolerance and Sandostatin

Tables 1 and 2 give the 24-h levels of blood glucose and serum insulin at 3 points of time during the study, i.e. before treatment was started, after about 4 months' therapy when 250 μg was given in 4 daily injections, and after about one year when the patients had received the highest dose: 500 μg t.i.d. for one month.

The diurnal blood glucose was initially

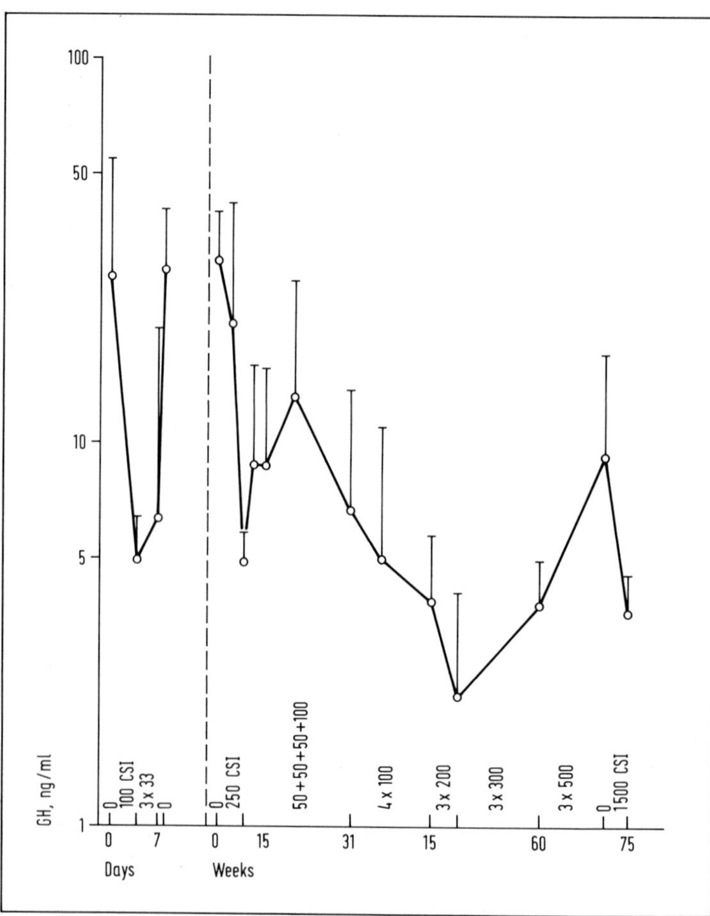

Fig. 1. Sandostatin (μg) administration schedule and serum growth hormone (GH) levels in one acromegalic patient. Sandostatin was given either as 3 or 4 daily injections, or as continuous subcutaneous infusion (CSI)

normal in all patients, a slight but significant decrease was observed at the second examination, while unchanged 24-h levels were noted at the end of the study when the patients received 500 μg Sandostatin t.i.d.

While it is beyond doubt that somatostatin and Sandostatin acutely suppress insulin release, we feel that the surprisingly well-preserved uniform and normal 24-h blood glucose later in this study strongly points to

Table 1. Change in 24-h blood glucose (mmol/l ± SD) at two different daily Sandostatin doses

Patient No.	Baseline	250 μg	1500 μg
301	5.63 ± 0.66	5.61 ± 1.28	5.60 ± 0.83
302	5.63 ± 0.83	5.03 ± 1.14	5.25 ± 0.84
303	5.76 ± 0.46	5.63 ± 1.24	5.97 ± 0.87
304	6.13 ± 0.84	5.54 ± 1.27	5.37 ± 0.90
306	5.60 ± 0.81	5.28 ± 1.17	5.51 ± 1.14
307	5.10 ± 0.46	4.86 ± 0.71	5.56 ± 0.84
308	4.90 ± 0.60	4.76 ± 0.90	4.95 ± 0.84
309	5.64 ± 0.85	5.20 ± 1.12	5.07 ± 0.74
310	6.13 ± 0.84	5.60 ± 0.92	5.87 ± 0.61
311	5.30 ± 0.58	5.16 ± 0.93	5.74 ± 0.74
Mean ± SD	5.58 ± 0.40	5.27 ± 0.32	5.49 ± 0.33

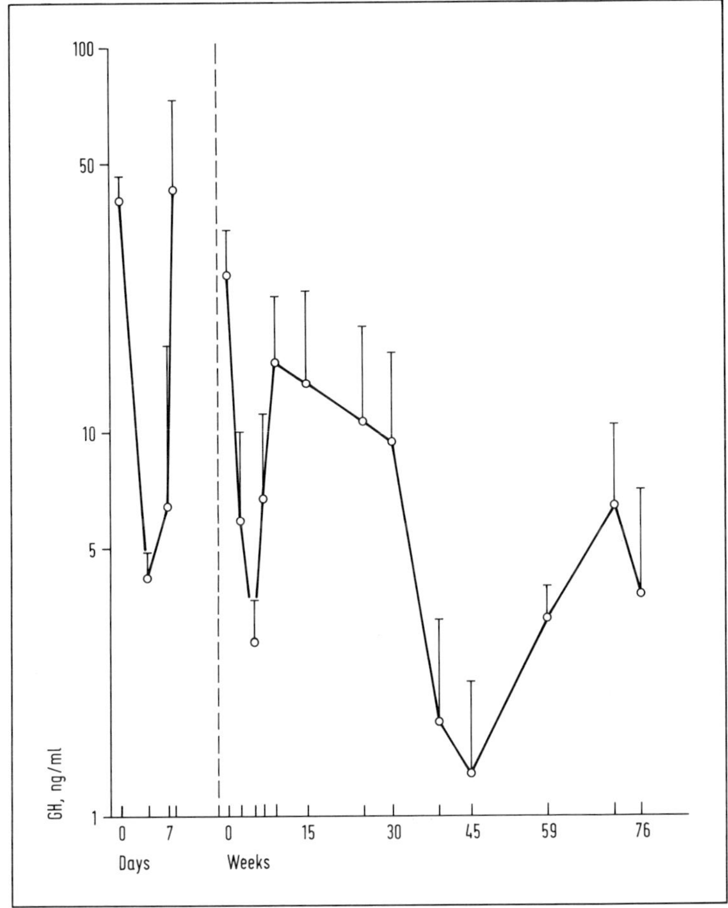

Fig. 2. Sandostatin administration as in Figure 1 in another acromegalic patient

a sustained ability to release insulin in accord with requirements. This impression is strengthened by observation of the changes in 24-h serum insulin concentrations, which declined markedly in all patients but one. However, those five patients (Nos 303; 306; 308; 310; 311) who had 24-h GH levels above 9 ng/ml at the final examination did not achieve the low 24-h serum insulin levels seen in the other five patients with pre-

Table 2. Change in 24-h serum insulin (μU/ml $\pm$ SD) at two different daily Sandostatin doses

Patient No.	Baseline	250 μg	1500 μg
301	45.2 $\pm$ 30.3	41.4 $\pm$ 19.8	24.6 $\pm$ 12.3
302	57.3 $\pm$ 44.9	37.5 $\pm$ 7.9	25.2 $\pm$ 13.4
303	20.4 $\pm$ 12.0	19.6 $\pm$ 12.4	24.7 $\pm$ 30.9
304	14.4 $\pm$ 19.5	20.4 $\pm$ 15.6	2.6 $\pm$ 3.2
306	30.6 $\pm$ 19.2	34.6 $\pm$ 14.0	34.6 $\pm$ 18.2
307	35.2 $\pm$ 16.3	13.3 $\pm$ 7.5	14.0 $\pm$ 9.0
308	39.9 $\pm$ 13.6	45.7 $\pm$ 11.5	32.7 $\pm$ 12.5
309	48.1 $\pm$ 46.0	26.5 $\pm$ 12.1	13.0 $\pm$ 11.7
310	48.2 $\pm$ 29.7	36.5 $\pm$ 18.6	30.4 $\pm$ 24.8
311	44.5 $\pm$ 23.1	22.5 $\pm$ 19.7	33.1 $\pm$ 28.6
Mean $\pm$ SD	38.4 $\pm$ 13.4	29.8 $\pm$ 10.8	23.5 $\pm$ 10.5

sumed lower insulin resistance − or had minimal reduction from the initial value.

In conclusion, prolonged Sandostatin administration does not seem to prevent appropriate insulin secretion in acromegalic patients. This is in accord with the tendency of some endocrine and other 'side effects' of Sandostatin to be transient after initiation of administration or after augmentation of dosage. In contrast, Sandostatin's effect on growth hormone release seems to be unimpaired during long-term administration.

Relationship between Serum Sandostatin Levels, its Metabolism and its Effect on Serum Growth Hormone

We had the opportunity to evaluate 24-h serum Sandostatin and GH during the several different Sandostatin administrations. Figure 3 illustrates the profiles in one patient at the highest and lowest dosage of 33 µg and 500 µg t.i.d. Note the different ordinates. During low-dose administration serum Sandostatin elevations to about 600 pg/ml suppressed serum GH from about 25

to 1 ng/ml; this occurred after each of the 3 subcutaneous injections. During injections of 500 µg, serum growth hormone showed similar undulations albeit with half as large an amplitude. Serum growth hormone thus rose in spite of serum Sandostatin levels, which were always several-fold higher than the effectively suppressive peak concentrations obtaining during 33 µg t.i.d.

One explanation for this phenomenon may be down regulation of a number of somatostatin receptor sites in the adenoma. The log-linear serum disappearance curves are well suited for evaluation of "serum half-lives", which were consistently about 100 min in this patient after subcutaneous injection of 33 µg and about 200 min after 500 µg. Since a sizeable fraction of somatostatin degradation probably takes place after binding to specific receptors, and these are presumed present in many tissues, the decreased Sandostatin degradation may also be an indicator of universal somatostatin receptor down regulation after treatment with large amounts of Sandostatin.

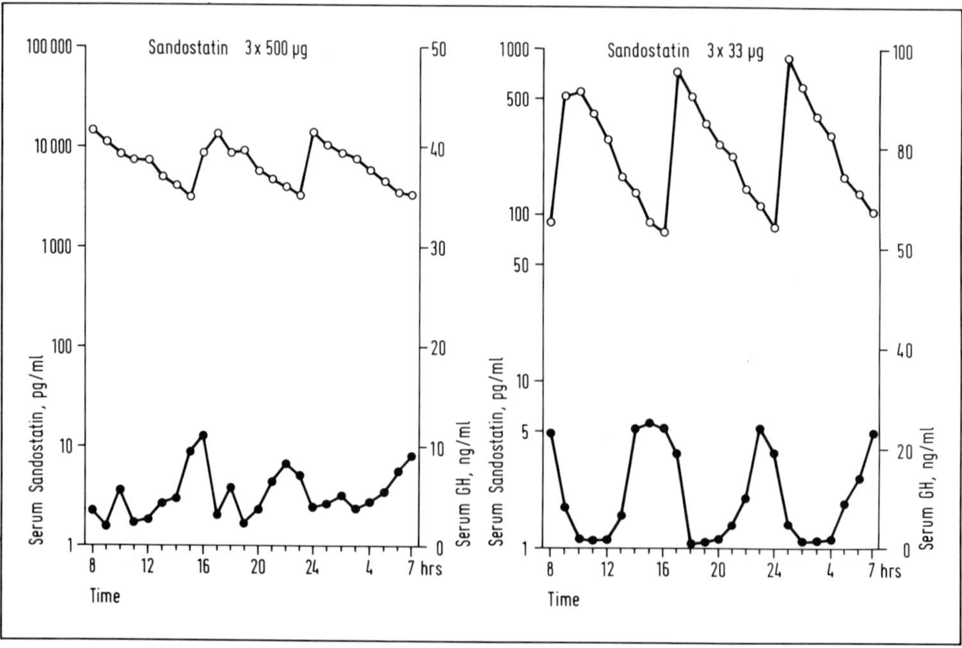

Fig. 3. 24-h serum growth hormone (●) and Sandostatin (○) (log scale) during 33 µg and 500 µg Sandostatin t.i.d. in one acromegalic patient

Acknowledgements: The technical assistance of Kirsten Nyborg, Lone Korsgaard, Inga Bisgaard, Pia Nielsen and Ninna Rosenqvist is gratefully acknowledged. We are also grateful to Dr. J. Rosenthaler, Sandoz, Basle, for gifts of excellent material for Sandostatin radioimmunoassay.

Reference

1. Christensen SE, Weeke J, Ørskov H, Møller N, Flyvbjerg A, Harris AG, Lund E, Jørgensen J (1987) Continuous subcutaneous pump infusion of somatostatin analogue SMS 201-995 versus subcutaneous injection schedule in acromegalic patients. Clin Endocrinol 27: 297−306

12. Effects of Long-Term Administration of Sandostatin® (SMS 201-995) at Increasing Doses in 40 Acromegalic Patients. Results from the French Sandostatin Acromegaly Study Group*

G. Sassolas[1], P. Fossati, P. Chanson, R. Costa, B. Estour, A. Deidier[2], A. G. Harris[3]

[1] Centre de Médecine Nucléaire, Lyon, France, [2] Recherches Cliniques, Sandoz, Rueil Malmaison, France, [3] Clinical Research, Sandoz Ltd, Basle, Switzerland

Several studies demonstrate the efficacy of short- and long-term Sandostatin® treatment in acromegaly administered subcutaneously at doses ranging from 150 to 300 µg up to 600 µg per day [1, 3, 5, 7–10]. A rhythm of 3 injections per day has been shown to reduce the magnitude of the re-elevation of growth hormone (GH) which occurs before the following injection when Sandostatin is given only twice daily. However, some patients fail to respond adequately to the above-mentioned doses thus pointing to the possible need for higher doses of Sandostatin [1] or continuous subcutaneous infusion.

To address this issue, the French Sandostatin Acromegaly Study Group performed a multicenter, prospective, open label trial of thrice daily injections of Sandostatin at increasing doses, with the aim of normalizing GH secretion and possibly achieving pituitary tumor size reduction.

Patients and Methods

Forty patients with acromegaly, informed of what the protocol involved, agreed to

take part in the trial, previously approved by our Institutional Ethics Committee. Active acromegaly was assessed clinically and biochemically (defined as mean GH plasma levels >5 µg/l). There were 23 women, aged 29–72 years (mean: 50.9 years) and 17 men, aged 22–71 years (mean: 48 years).

In twenty-nine patients, the pituitary tumor had been removed and subsequently treated by external radiotherapy. Sandostatin was given as primary treatment to eleven patients either because they were too old or because they presented cardiovascular disorders contraindicating surgery and could not await the improvement following radiotherapy.

In some cases, the size of the tumors, their localization or their expansion, for instance into the cavernous sinus, suggested that satisfactory tumor removal of the adenoma could not be expected.

Investigations before inclusion in the protocol included hourly measurements of plasma GH levels during a 12–24-h period and oral glucose load (75 g) and Sm-C radioimmunoassay. Pituitary tumor evaluations (ophthalmological examination and CT scan) were also performed. Sandostatin treatment was initiated in hospital, starting with 3 injections of 50 µg per day increasing two days later to 100 µg × 3. Sandostatin doses were increased at monthly intervals as follows: 100 µg × 3, 200 µg × 3, 300 µg × 3, 500 µg × 3. Sandostatin dosage was to be increased if GH levels were not normalized (defined as 75% of GH values below the level of detectability for usual assays). Treatment was continued for a further three months on the maximum dose for each patient. At the end of this period, in addition

* Participating Centers:
P. Allanic, Y. Lorcy/Rennes, B. Charbonnel/Nantes, P. Fossati, D. Dewailly, O. Verrier-Mine/Lille, Ph. Jacquet/Marseille, J. P. Louvet, A. Bennet/Toulouse, J. Lubetzki, Ph. Chanson, J. Timsit, A. Warnet/Paris, J. Mirouze, M. Rodier/Montpellier, H. Rousset, B. Estour/St. Etienne, G. Sassolas, J. P. Casez, P. Serusclat/Lyon, M. Simon, G. Edan, J. P. Hespel/Rennes Trial coordination: A. G. Harris (Basle), A. Deidier (Rueil-Malmaison)

to the usual tolerability and efficacy evaluation, an ophthalmological examination, CT scan and ultrasonography of the biliary tract were performed.

Eighteen patients reached the maximum dose of 500 μg × 3, nine patients reached 300 μg × 3, five reached 200 μg × 3 and six remained on 100 μg × 3. All patients self-injected Sandostatin.

Results

As some parameters concerning tolerability and efficacy have not yet been fully analysed, the results reported here are to be considered preliminary.

Tolerability

Four patients out of forty dropped out of the trial; two of them experienced abdominal pain and severe diarrhea at the onset of treatment.

The third patient experienced the same symptoms during the third month of treatment. The fourth patient while on 300 μg × 3 complained of acute abdominal pain during the sixth month of treatment, leading to withdrawal. Ten days later a melena occurred, the origin of which could not be determined. It is noteworthy that this patient had previously undergone surgery for a non-secreting endocrine pancreatic tumor.

Fifteen patients complained of intermittent diarrhea and 25 of loose stools at some stage during treatment, particularly at the beginning or when the dose was increased. Abdominal pain was noted in 9 patients and nausea in 4. These symptoms did not lead to treatment interruption.

In three patients, asymptomatic gallstones appeared during the treatment, detected on ultrasonography. Reduced hemoglobin levels and red cell count was noted in 14 patients. In two cases, this could be accounted for by the melena mentioned above and by silent digestive bleeding. In the other cases, no explanation could be found for the gradual decline in hemoglobin and red cell count other than the repeated blood sampling required to perform the 12−14-h GH profile. Moreover, it should be noted that blood indices normalized spontaneously during Sandostatin therapy when blood sampling was done less frequently.

Carbohydrate Tolerance

Carbohydrate tolerance was assessed on diurnal, hourly determinations of blood glucose and insulin before treatment and on each dose. Mean blood glucose values (± SD) did not vary significantly: 6.5 ± 1.9 (pretreatment), 6.4 ± 1 (100 μg × 3), 6.5 ± 1 (200 μg × 3), 6.8 ± 2.8 (300 μg × 3), 7.1 ± 2 mmol/l (500 μg × 3), despite a 23 to 25% decrease of plasma insulin concentrations compared with pretreatment levels. Moreover these variations were not dose-related. The oral glucose administration at the end of the protocol, on the maximum Sandostatin dose, induced higher glucose and lower insulin levels than pretreatment values in the same subjects (Fig. 1).

Clinical Improvement

In 34 out of 38 patients analysed, Sandostatin treatment resulted in rapid clinical improvement, on the lowest dose. The decrease in soft tissue swelling was probably responsible for the initial weight loss (mean: 3 kg), comparable to that observed after successful surgical removal of adenoma in acromegaly. Excessive perspiration was rapidly reduced in most patients. Paresthesias which had been noted before treatment in 6 patients disappeared in 2 of them. Headache, present in 21 patients, was markedly ameliorated in 7 patients, partially reduced in 13, unchanged in 1 patient. Some patients described a clear relationship between the symptomatic effect and the Sandostatin dose. In two patients for whom heart transplantation had been envisaged, cardiac insufficiency, considered to be related to acromegaly, was dramatically improved during the first weeks of treatment, thus avoiding surgery. One patient suffering from sleep apnea showed dramatic improvement [2]. Fourteen patients suffered from depression before treatment. Marked amelioration occurred in eight. In one patient who dropped out for digestive symptoms, depression appeared to worsen.

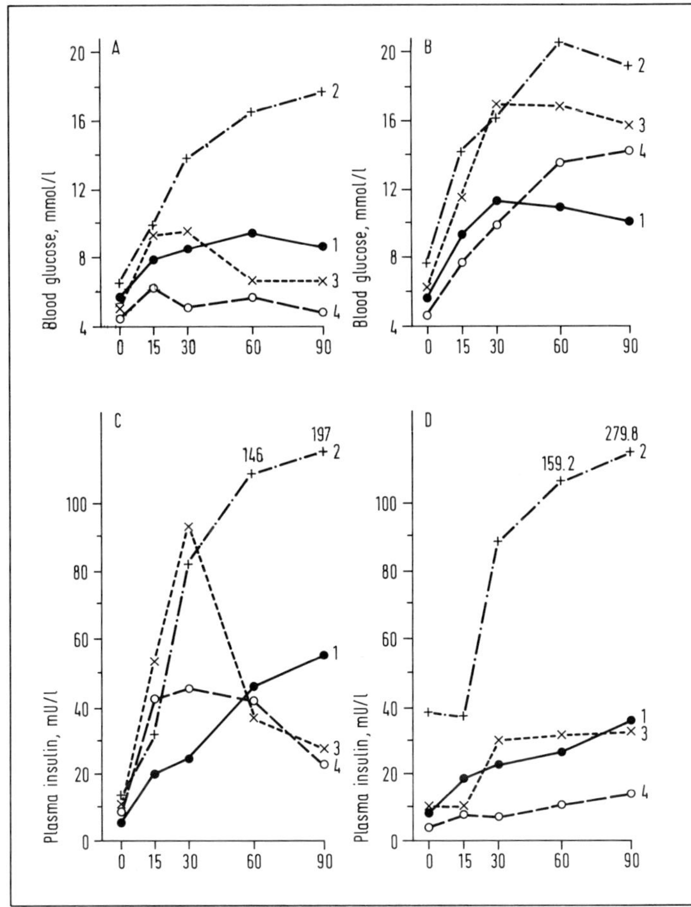

Fig. 1. Effects on glucose and insulin plasma concentration during a 75 g glucose test performed in 4 patients before and at the 6th month of Sandostatin treatment. A and C indicate the values before treatment, B and D the values during treatment

Effects on GH Secretion

The protocol included 12–24 GH profiles which have not yet been thoroughly evaluated. For instance, the number of normalized profiles cannot, at present, be given. Therefore, only mean GH concentrations are provided. Figure 2 shows individual values of mean GH concentration for each dose. The averages of the mean plasma concentrations ($\pm$ SD) were 21.4 $\pm$ 27 µg/l before treatment, 7 $\pm$ 8 µg/l (100 µg $\times$ 3), 6.4 $\pm$ 5.7 µg/l (200 µg $\times$ 3), 6.9 $\pm$ 6.3 µg/l (300 µg $\times$ 3) and 6.8 $\pm$ 4.4 µg/l /(500 µg $\times$ 3). The mean GH reduction was 43, 53, 51 and 61% on the four doses respectively. The difference between mean GH concentrations before Sandostatin therapy and all four doses, compared by 2-way analysis of variance, in the 18 patients who received the four doses was found to be significant (0.005 $< p < 0.01$). Multiple comparisons showed a significant difference between 100 µg $\times$ 3 and 500 µg $\times$ 3 (0.01 $< p < 0.025$).

The percentage of GH reduction achieved by 100 µg $\times$ 3 strongly correlated with the mean pretreatment concentration. If a mean GH concentration lower than 50% of the mean pretreatment value is considered as a criterion of efficacy, it appears that the percentage of profiles reaching this limit did not differ significantly from one dose to another (Fig. 3). Four patients (irrespective of Sandostatin dose) failed to reduce their GH levels to below 50% of the pretreatment value. This data is confirmed by the distribution of mean GH concentration (Fig. 4) showing that five patients had mean GH values higher than 10 µg/l during treatment on the maximum Sandostatin

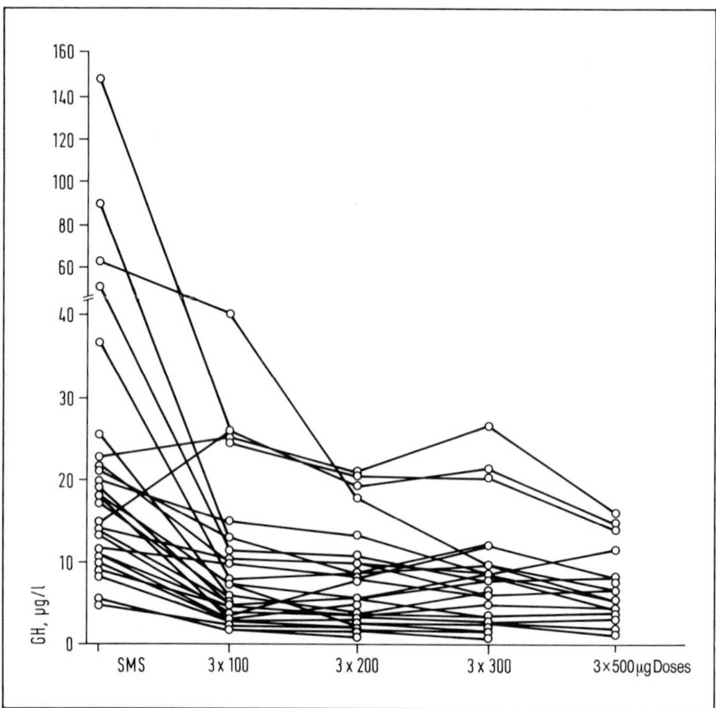

Fig. 2. Individual values of mean plasma growth hormone (GH) levels evaluated before and during the treatment at different doses. *SMS* (Sandostatin)

dose and twenty-three reached GH mean values below 5 µg/l, twelve of them with values equal to or less than 2 µg/l.

In this trial, during which all subjects did not receive all four doses, the data show that the optimal dose is 100 µg × 3 in eighteen patients, 200 µg × 3 in eight patients, 300 µg × 3 in four and 500 µg × 3 in eight.

On the highest dose, the difference in GH reduction was minimal in five patients out of eight. The data suggest a slight dose-response relationship above 100 µg × 3 in eight patients only. No further benefit could be noted by increasing the dose in 13/18 patients.

Sm-C/IGFI

Overall analysis of the Sm-C data is not yet available, since different radioimmunoassays were used at the various study centers. However, according to the reference values for each assay, Sm-C levels normalized on Sandostatin treatment in 17/31 patients for whom this information is now available.

Effects on Tumor Volume

Only 27 cases can be analysed at the present time. Tumor reduction of 20−50% was observed in 7 cases and a reduction greater than 50% in 3 tumors with suprasellar extension. These three patients received the maximum dose (500 µg × 3), which produced a dramatic reduction in mean GH values.

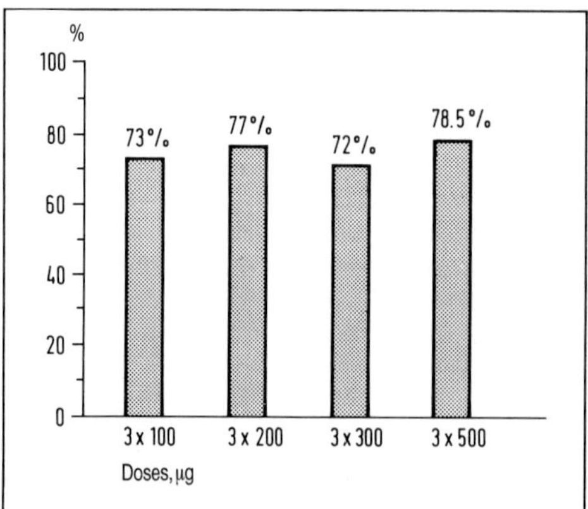

Fig. 3. Percentages of GH profiles with mean GH levels below 50% of the pretreatment values

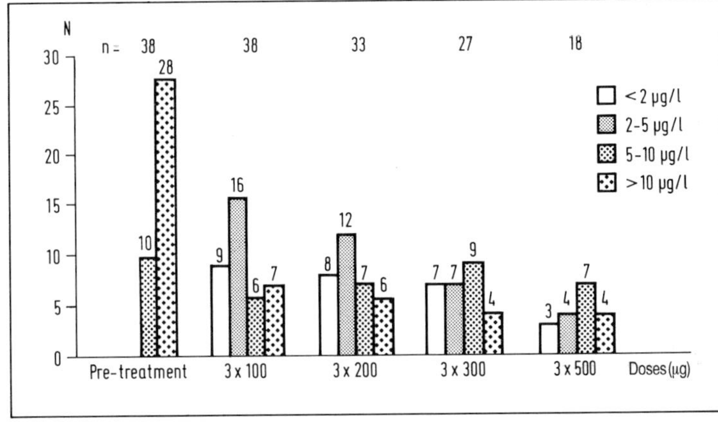

Fig. 4. Distribution of mean GH levels according to four different classes on different Sandostatin doses

Discussion

The data reported here show that Sandostatin provides clinical improvement in the majority of our patients (34 out of 40). Only four patients dropped out of the study. Gastrointestinal side effects experienced by some of the other patients did not lead to treatment interruption. The occurrence of gallstones, the incidence of which cannot be fully evaluated at the present time, gave us cause for concern.

Such a complication had been previously reported with Sandostatin treatment in a patient with a TSH-producing adenoma [4].

Acromegalic patients undergoing Sandostatin therapy should, therefore, be carefully evaluated by ultrasonography and cholecystography.

In overall terms, 23 out of 38 patients achieved a mean GH concentration equal to or lower than 5 µg/l and 12 of them a mean concentration equal to or lower than 2 µg/l, which may be considered a good result. Four patients failed to respond to Sandostatin treatment despite our policy of increasing doses. This may be related to the low density of somatostatin receptors.

Increasing Sandostatin doses further reduced GH levels in some cases. However, in the majority of our acromegalic patients, dose increments did not modify the results. The data obtained from the present collection of patients suggests that the optimal Sandostatin dose is 100 µg three times daily. Tumor size reduction was obtained in approximately 25% of patients. Since the study did not require repeated CT scans on the different doses, it is not possible to assess how fast tumor size reduction was achieved and on which dose.

In line with a recent editorial in the New England Journal of Medicine [6] Sandostatin may be considered an effective new treatment for acromegaly. This disease has led many physicians to despair.

Most patients feel a remarkable improvement. Ten per cent fail to respond. The constraints of Sandostatin treatment are that it must be administered subcutaneously three times daily. However, other routes are currently under consideration. At present the indications for Sandostatin in acromegalic patients are the failure of surgical and radiotherapy treatment or their contraindications. This new medical approach enables the practitioner to be less passive in the management of this disease.

References

1. Barnard LG, Grantham WG, Lamberton P, O'Dorisio TM, Jackson IMD (1986) Treatment of resistant acromegaly with a long-acting Somatostatin analogue (SMS 201-995). Ann Intern Med 105:856–861
2. Chanson P, Timsit J, Benoit O, Augendre B, Boulonguet M, Guillausseau PJ, Warnet A, Lubetzki J (1968) Rapid improvement in sleep apnoea of acromegaly after short-term treatment with somatostatin analogue SMS 201-995. Lancet ii:1270–1271
3. Ch'ng LJC, Sandler LM, Kraenzlin ME, Burin JM, Joplin CF, Bloom SR (1985)

Long-term treatment of acromegaly with a long-acting analogue of somatostatin. Br Med J 290:284−288

4. Comi RJ, Gesundheit N, Murray L, Gorden P, Weintraub BD (1987) Response of thyrotropin-secreting pituitary adenomas to a long-acting somatostatin analogue. N Engl J Med 317:12−17

5. Comi RJ, Gorden P (1987) The response of serum growth hormone levels to the long-acting somatostatin analog SMS 201-995 in acromegaly. J Clin Endocrinol Metab 64: 37−42

6. Daughaday W (1985) A new treatment for an old disease. N Engl J Med 313:1604−1605

7. Lamberts SWJ, Oosterom R, Neufeld M, Del Pozo E (1985) The somatostatin analog SMS 201-995 induces long-acting inhibition of growth hormone secretion without re-bound hypersecretion in acromegalic patients. J Clin Endocrinol Metab 60: 1161−1170

8. Lamberts SJ, Uitterlinden P, Del Pozo E (1987) SMS 201-995 induces a continuous decline in circulating growth hormone and somatomedin-C levels during therapy of acromegaly for over two years. J Clin Endocrinol Metab 65:703−710

9. Lamberts SWJ, Uitterlinden P. Verschoor L, van Dongen KJ, Del Pozo E (1985) Long-term treatment of acromegaly with the somatostatin analogue SMS 201-995. N Engl J Med 313:1576− 1580

10. Plewe G, Beyer J, Krause U, Neufeld M, Del Pozo E (1984) Long-acting and selective suppression of growth hormone secretion by somatostatin analogue SMS 201-995 in acromegaly. Lancet II:782−784

13. Experience with Sandostatin® in Various Groups of Acromegalic Patients

A. Stevenaert[1], A. Beckers[1], K. Kovacs[1], E. Bastings[1], M. de Longueville[2], G. Hennen[1]

[1]Universities of Liège, Belgium, and Toronto, Canada and [2]Sandoz, Brussels, Belgium

The availability, for clinical use, of the somatostatin analogue SMS 201-995 (Sandostatin®) has opened new doors in the treatment of acromegaly [1, 5, 6]. We report here our experience with Sandostatin used either as a chronic medical therapy or as a preparation to surgery.

Patients and Methods

Twenty-eight acromegalic patients (16 men and 12 women; age 24.2−68.0 years) were divided into three groups: *Group I* comprised 12 unselected patients treated for 3 to 6 weeks with subcutaneous injection of Sandostatin 100 µg t.i.d. until transsphenoidal adenomectomy. *Group II* was composed of 8 patients without any previous treatment and for whom a 6-month Sandostatin therapy prior to surgery was planned. Sandostatin dosage was increased from a starting dose of 300 µg to a maximum dose of 1500 µg per day. *Group III* included 11 patients with unsuccessful previous treatment, or recurrence (from whom two cases were recruited from Group I and one from Group II). In this group, dose adjustment depended on tolerability and therapeutic efficacy with a maximum dosage of 1500 µg per day in 10 cases and 3000 µg in the last one.

In all three groups, clinical, biological and radiological parameters were monitored. Growth hormone (GH) diurnal profiles and basal somatomedin-C (Sm-C) values were determined before treatment and at different intervals during treatment. CT scans of the sella turcica were perfomed before treatment and after 3 weeks in Group I and 6 months in Group II. In vitro cultures of adenomas were obtained in 10 cases from Group I (K. Mashiter, Hammersmith Hospital, London).

Clinical Results

Out of 28 patients, clinical results were excellent (disappearance of all complaints and decrease in soft tissue swelling) in 15 cases and good (disappearance of some complaints or signs and diminution of the others) in 7 cases. In the 19 chronically treated patients (Table 1) the rate of clinical remission was 73.7%. The patients from Groups I and III exhibited similar results in both protocols: excellent in one, nil in the other. One other patient had poor results on Group II protocol while she was more responsive with Group III protocol, i.e. Sandostatin after surgery.

Biological Results

In Group I patients, mean GH values were significantly decreased after the first injection. Figure 1 shows the diurnal GH profiles before and during Sandostatin treatment in one case. Mean GH values were under 5 ng/ml in 5 patients after 1 week and in 8 patients after 3 weeks of treatment. Sm-C levels were also reduced in all patients and normalized in 5 patients within 3 weeks. After transsphenoidal adenomectomy, GH levels were under 5 ng/ml and Sm-C levels were within normal limits in 9 out of 12 patients.

Biological results in Groups II and III are illustrated in Figures 2 and 3. Normalization of GH values (i.e. level equal to or below 5 ng/ml) occurred in 5 patients from Group

Table 1. Clinical results with long-term Sandostatin treatment (Group II, cases 1–8; Group III, cases 9–19)

Cases	Previous operation	Previous radio-therapy	Sandostatin µg/day	Duration of treatment (months)	Clinical results
1	−	−	1500	6	Poor
2	−	−	1500	6	Poor
3	−	−	900	6	Excellent
4	−	−	1500	9	Poor
5	−	−	600	3	Good
6	−	−	600	2	Excellent
7	−	−	600	6	Good
8	−	−	900	2	Good
9	+	+	3000	12	Nil
10	+	+	900	9	Excellent
11	+	+	1500	11	Good
12	+	+	1500	11	Good
13	+	+	900	10	Excellent
14	+	+	600	22	Excellent
15	+	+	1500	5	Good
16	+	−	600	2	Good
17	+	−	300	3	Excellent
18	+	−	300	6	Excellent
19	−	+	600	5	Poor

II and 9 patients from Group III (73.7% of the cases). At the 2 ng/ml level, 6 patients (31.6%) had GH profiles within this limit. Sm-C levels were decreased in all patients and normalized in 12 patients (63.2%).

Radiological and Pathological Data

Among the 12 patients in Group I, 5 showed slight pituitary tumor size reduction, while in a sixth case, the vertical diameter of the tumor was reduced by 33%. In 3 patients from Group II treated with Sandostatin for 6 months no significant change was observed. In Group III patients, changes due to surgery and/or radiotherapy did not allow any CT scan evaluation for comparison.

Tumor specimens obtained at operation were subjected to pathological studies. Few pathological changes were noted after Sandostatin treatment and consisted in widening of the perivascular space and more crinophagy than in untreated cases [Becker et al., to be published].

In vitro cultures of 10 Sandostatin-treated adenomas and 21 untreated tumors were performed by K. Mashiter (Hammersmith Hospital, London). The amounts of secreted GH (range: 100 to 1000 ng/200 000 cells/24 h) were similar in treated and in untreated cases.

Adverse Events

In our series, Sandostatin was well tolerated although some adverse events were observed. Pain at the site of injection, mild or moderate, was spontaneously reported by 20% of the patients.

Gastrointestinal adverse effects occurred in 20 out of the 28 patients (71.4%) and consisted usually in abdominal discomfort and transient diarrhea. In 2 patients, Sandostatin was discontinued due to the severity of diarrhea in one case and abdominal pain in the other.

In 10 patients, ultrasound examinations of gallbladder and biliary tract were performed prior to and after 6-month Sandostatin treatment, with an increasing dose regimen up to 1500 µg daily. Two patients developed asymptomatic gallstones.

The possibility of steatorrhea has not been investigated but assays of carotene,

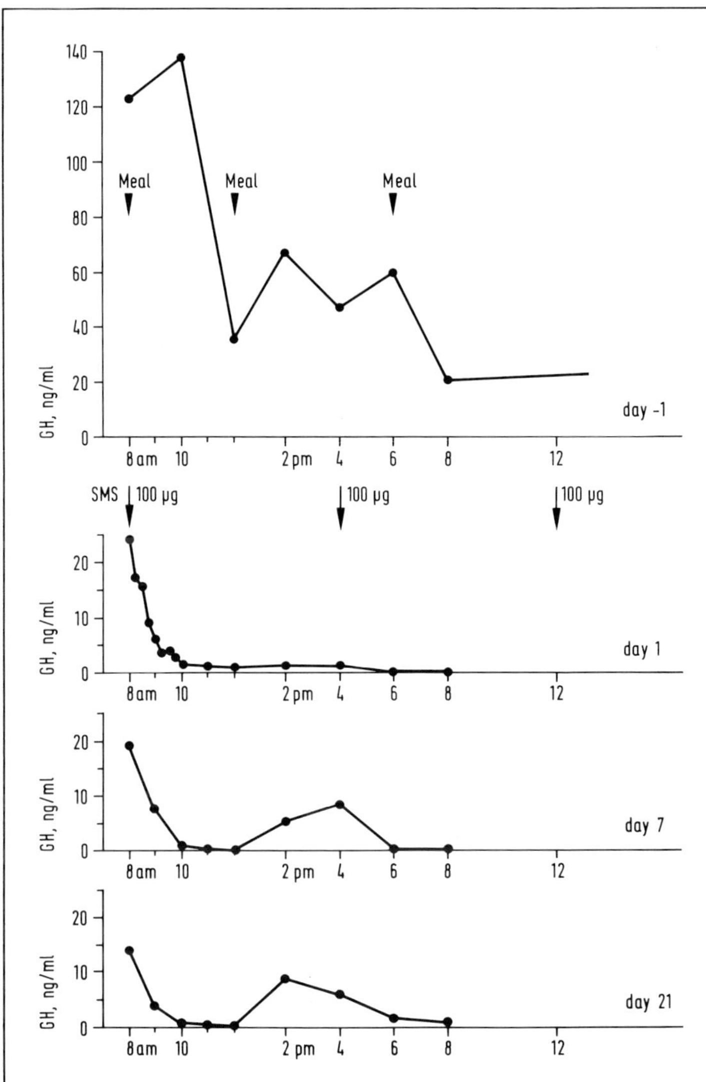

Fig. 1. Plasma growth hormone (GH) response to Sandostatin (SMS) 100 µg t.i.d. Diurnal GH profiles are shown before treatment (day − 1) and on day 1, day 7 and day 21

vitamin A and vitamin D were performed in order to determine possible malabsorption. Most patients exhibited a decrease in carotene values during the first months of treatment and, in 9 cases, the levels fell below the lower normal limit of 0.6 ng/ml at a given time of treatment (Fig. 4). The decrease was transient in some cases but more persistent in others. No significant change was observed in vitamin A studies (Fig. 5), except in one patient in whom vitamin A levels fell from 4.7 to 3.0 mIU/l while simultaneously carotene levels fell from 1.1 to 0.2 ng/ml; moreover, in this case Sandostatin was discontinued due to the severity of diarrhea. Vitamin D studies (Fig. 6) showed no significant change of values during treatment. Carbohydrate metabolism was also monitored during treatment. Fasting blood glucose values remained unchanged as did glycosylated hemoglobin (Fig. 7) except in one diabetic patient who showed a decrease from 12% to 6.8%, without any change in insulin dosage. In the other cases, glycosylated hemoglobin remained within the normal limits.

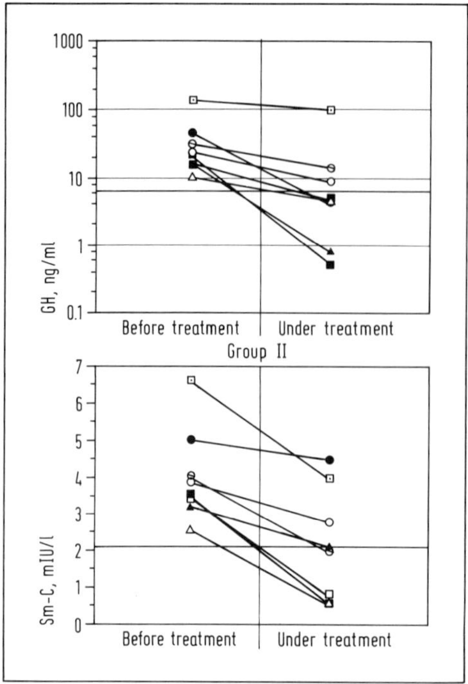

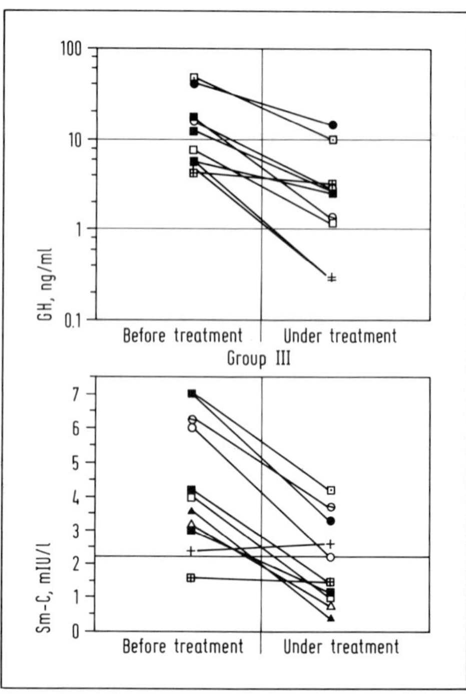

Fig. 2. Mean growth hormone (GH) and basal somatomedin-C (Sm-C) values in Group II patients before and during Sandostatin treatment

Fig. 3. Mean GH and basal Sm-C values in Group III patients before and on Sandostatin treatment

Discussion

Treatment of acromegaly remains a difficult challenge and until recently it was based on transsphenoidal surgery and conventional radiotherapy. The goal of treatment is to achieve clinical cure and normalization of GH and Sm-C values. Although the term

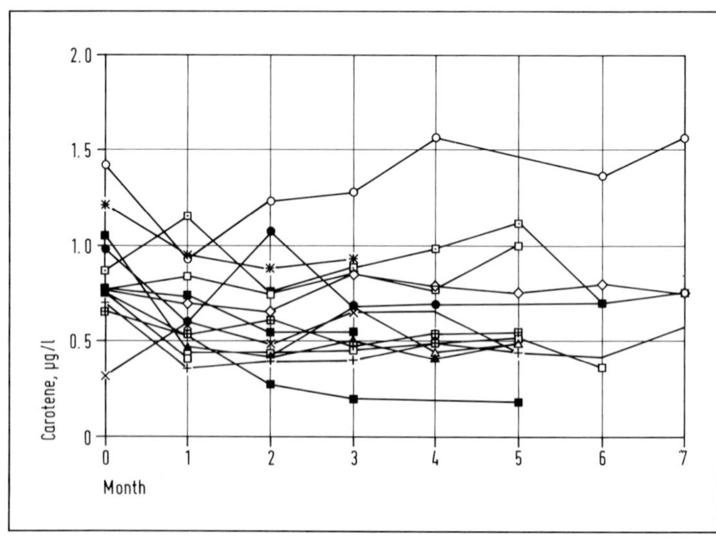

Fig. 4. Carotene values (N = 0.6 − 2.4 µg/l) in 16 patients on Sandostatin treatment

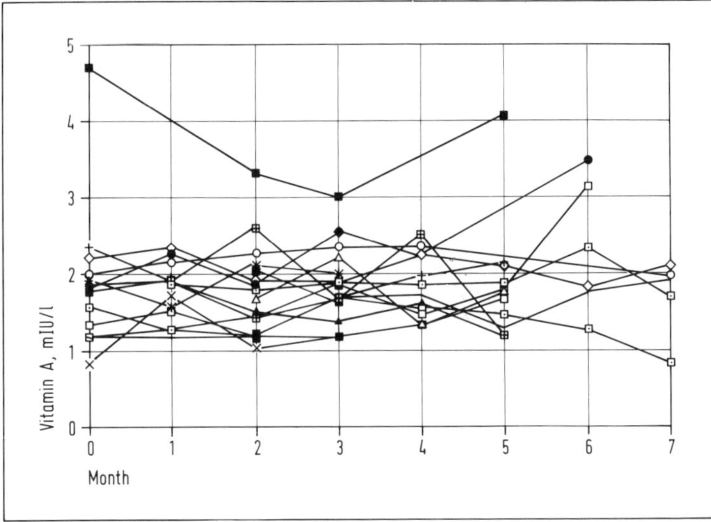

Fig. 5. Vitamin A values (N = 1.0 − 2.0 mIU/l) in 17 patients on Sandostatin treatment

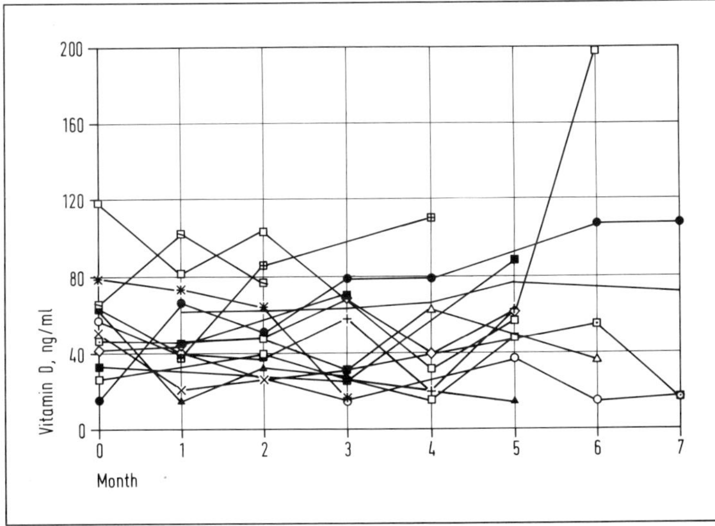

Fig. 6. Vitamin D values (N = 15 − 88 ng/ml) in 16 patients on Sandostatin treatment

"cure" is generally agreed, the concept of "remission" seems more satisfactory to evaluate therapeutic results. Normalization of GH is also equivocal and different levels are accepted. We considered as normalization a cut-off level of 5 ng/ml although it could be situated lower still. So defined, the overall "remission" rate was 68.3% in 104 operated acromegalic patients with a range of 90% in enclosed adenomas and 48% in invasive macroadenomas.

The GH suppressive effect of Sandostatin and its advantages in acromegaly treatment were recently established [5−7]. In this study, Sandostatin was administered to three different groups of patients.

Short-term administration of Sandostatin 100 µg t.i.d. normalized GH diurnal profiles in 8 patients out of 12. However, Sm-C values decreased within normal limits in only 5 cases. To achieve better results, it may be necessary to increase Sandostatin doses or treatment duration. Nevertheless it is noteworthy that successful transsphenoi-

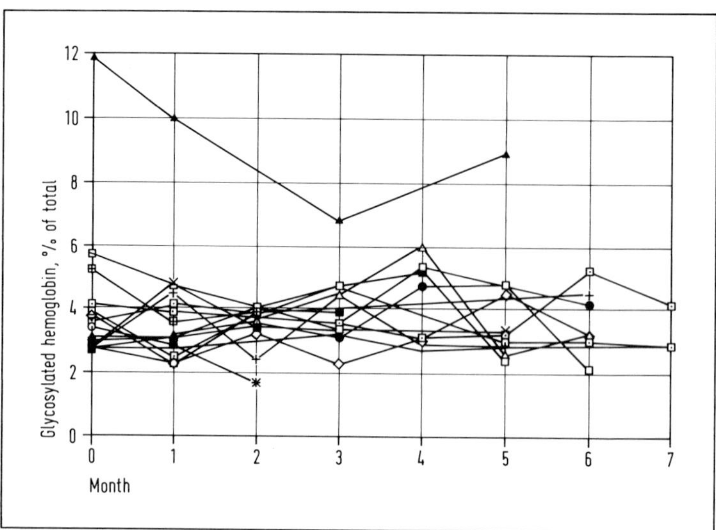

Fig. 7. Glycosylated hemoglobin levels (N < 6.5%) in 17 patients on Sandostatin treatment

dal surgery achieved Sm-C normalization within a few days in 9 out of the 12 patients. In long-term Sandostatin-treated patients, normalization of GH values was achieved in 73.7% of the cases while Sm-C was within normal limits in only 63.2% in line with clinical results.

Tumor shrinkage could be an additional indication of therapeutic efficacy though, in our series, significant changes only occurred in one case while some others exhibited only slight tumor size reduction [4, 9]. In our experience Sandostatin does not seem to be very effective in reducing adenoma size and these data are in line with our pathological findings and in vitro culture results. It could be that Sandostatin acts preferentially on GH release rather than on synthesis.

Tolerability of Sandostatin was usually good. The more frequent adverse effects consisted of transient gastrointestinal disturbances lasting for a few days but occurring again at every increase in dosage regimen. Only in 2 cases was Sandostatin discontinued owing to the severity of such gastrointestinal side effects. 2 patients developed asymptomatic gallstones.

Our results of carotene plasma level determinations suggest possible fat malabsorption in some cases. Long-term Sandostatin treatment requires adequate monitoring so that supplemental therapy be given as required.

Carbohydrate metabolism did not deteriorate as monitored by fasting glucose levels and glycosylated hemoglobin determinations. Furthermore, in diabetic patients, glucose metabolism improved possibly because of GH suppression.

In conclusion, Sandostatin proved effective in improving the clinical condition in acromegalic patients as well as their hormonal parameters. In long-term treatment the remission rate was 70%. The optimal dosage ranged from 300 to 900 µg daily with good tolerability although some adverse effects may occur, such as gallstone formation and malabsorption. In spite of the clinical and biological efficacy of Sandostatin, mild or moderate tumor shrinkage occurred only in a few cases.

References

1. Bauer W, Briner U, Doepfner W et al. (1982) SMS 201-995: a very potent and selective octapeptide analogue of Somatostatin with prolonged action. Life Sci 31:1133
2. Beckers A, Stevenaert A, Hennen G (1987) Preoperative and long-term treatment of acromegaly with SMS 201-995. International Symposium on Growth Hormone Basic and Clinical Aspects, Tampa, Florida, June 1987 (abstract)
3. Beckers A, Stevenaert A, Hennen G (1987) SMS 201-995: Therapeutic indications for ac-

romegaly. First European Congress of Endocrinology, Copenhagen, 21−25 June, 1987 (abstract Nos 1−57)
4. Beckers A, Stevenaert A, de Longueville M, Thibaut A, Hennen G (1986) The treatment of acromegaly with the somatostatin analogue SMS 201-995. International Symposium Somatostatin, Madrid, 1986 (abstract)
5. Lamberts SWJ, Oosterom R, Neufeld M, Del Pozo E (1985) The somatostatin analog SMS 201-995 induces long-acting inhibition of growth hormone secretion without rebound hypersecretion in acromegalic patients. J Clin Endocrinol Metab 60:1161
6. Lamberts SWJ, Uitterlinden P, Verschoor L, van Dongen KJ, Del Pozo E (1985) Long-term treatment of acromegaly with the somatostatin analogue SMS 201-995. N Engl J Med 313:1576
7. Lamberts SWJ, Zweens M, Verschoor L, Del Pozo E (1986) A comparison among the growth hormone-lowering effects in acromegaly of the Somatostatin analog SMS 201-995, bromocriptine, and the combination of both drugs. J Clin Endocrinol Metab 63:16
8. Spinas GA, Zapf J, Landolt AM, Stuckmann G, Froesch ER (1987) Pre-operative treatment of 5 acromegalics with a somatostatin analogue: endocrine and clinical observations. Acta Endocrinol (Copenh) 114:249
9. Stevenaert A, Beckers A, Thibaut A, de Longueville M, Hennen G (1986) Preoperative treatment of acromegaly with SMS 201-995. Acromegaly Centennial Symposium, San Francisco, June 29−July 1 1986 (abstract P-18)

14. Treatment of Acromegaly with SMS 201-995 (Sandostatin®): Clinical, Biochemical and Morphologic Study

A. L. Barkan, R. V. Lloyd, W. F. Chandler, M. K. Hatfield, S. S. Gebarski, R. P. Kelch, I. Z. Beitins

Departments of Internal Medicine, Pathology, Surgery, Radiology and Pediatrics, Veterans Administration and University Hospitals, University of Michigan, Ann Arbor, Michigan, USA

Current therapy of acromegaly is unsatisfactory, and in a significant proportion of acromegalic patients the disease remains clinically active after all approved therapeutic modalities (surgery, irradiation and bromocriptine) have been exhausted.

Over the past 3 years, we have treated 21 acromegalic patients (twenty with pituitary tumors and one with pituitary somatotroph hyperplasia due to ectopic GHRH secretion from a metastatic carcinoid tumor) with somatostatin analog (SMS 201-995, Sandostatin®). Ten patients with pituitary tumors had been previously treated by surgery and irradiation, and some of them had also received bromocriptine, while another ten were newly-diagnosed and previously untreated. Results of Sandostatin therapy in 15 patients with pituitary tumors and in a patient with ectopic GHRH secretion have been reported elsewhere [1,2]. The protocol included the assessment of daily GH secretion (samples taken every 10 or 20 min for 24 h), measurement of somatomedin-C, assessment of GH responses to TRH (200 µg i.v.), GHRH 1-44 (1 µg/kg i.v.) and to bromocriptine (2.5 mg p.o.), as well as an oral glucose tolerance test (OGTT). A pituitary CT scan was done to assess the size and the invasiveness of the tumor. After that, the patients were placed on Sandostatin, 50–250 µg every 6 or 8 h s.c. Reassessment of GH secretory pattern was performed 5–7 days later, and patients continued Sandostatin therapy on an outpatient basis. Repeat inpatient assessment of GH secretion, and GH responsiveness to TRH, GHRH 1-44 as well as OGTT were performed 2 and 6 months later, and the patients were followed on an outpatient basis for up to 3 years. Ten newly-diagnosed patients underwent transsphenoidal or sub-frontal (in one) adenomectomy 3–30 weeks after initiation of Sandostatin therapy. Pituitary CT scan in these individuals was performed prior to surgery. The patient with ectopic GHRH secretion had extensive metastatic dissemination of the tumor (liver, lung, vertebrae, ribs, skull), and was previously treated with partial pituitary resection, pituitary irradiation, bromocriptine and chemotherapy (5-FU + streptozotocin). These modalities failed to suppress his GH hypersecretion (20–150 ng/ml), pituitary growth, plasma GHRH-LI (2–15 ng/ml; normal less than 0.05) or metastatic burden. In this patient, repeat estimates of plasma GH, Sm-C and GHRH-LI and pituitary and abdominal CT scans were repeated during a 3-year follow-up.

Results

Hormonal Responses

Eighteen of 20 patients with GH-producing pituitary tumors responded to Sandostatin therapy with a significant decrease (in 2), or normalization (in 16) of plasma GH and Sm-C. Clinical improvement became manifest after 2–4 days of Sandostatin therapy (Fig. 1). This was accompanied by the decrease in soft tissue hypertrophy, disappearance of excess perspiration and skin oiliness, and improved general well-being. In eight of nine patients exhibiting symptoms and signs of acromegalic arthropathy, joint complaints decreased significantly or disappeared altogether, and nerve entrapment symptoms (carpal tunnel syndrome) resolved. In two unresponsive patients, however, plasma GH remained elevated and

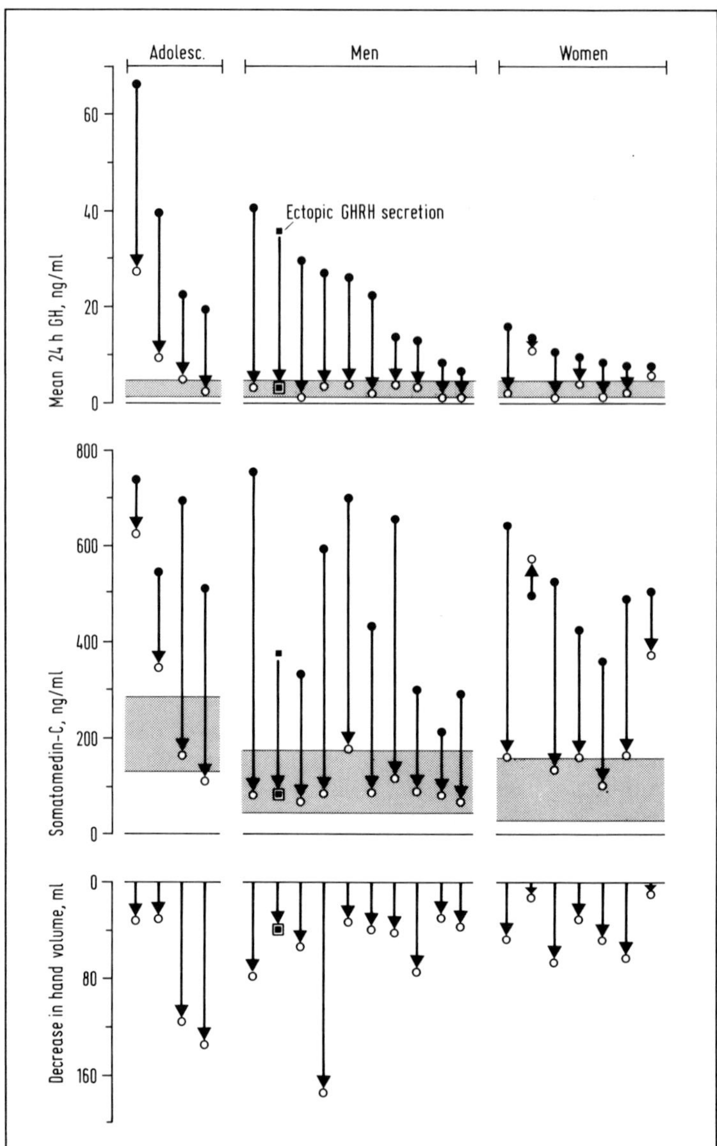

Fig. 1. Hormonal and clinical effects of long-term therapy with Sandostatin in patients with acromegaly. Solid circles represent values prior to Sandostatin therapy and open circles during Sandostatin therapy. Shaded areas mark normal ranges for mean 24-h plasma growth hormone (GH) and somatomedin-C. *GHRH* growth hormone releasing hormone

not even a transient decrease in plasma GH was evident on every 20 min blood sampling after each injection of Sandostatin. In one of them, the addition of bromocriptine (previously shown to be ineffective) resulted in a normalization of plasma GH and Sm-C concentrations and in a significant clinical improvement. Sandostatin completely suppressed plasma GH responses to GHRH 1-44, but only partial suppression of GH rises in response to TRH was noted (Fig. 2).

Plasma TSH responses to TRH and thyroid hormone concentrations were assessed in 15 patients not taking replacement thyroxine. A slight suppression of basal TSH, and approximately 50% inhibition of TSH responsiveness to TRH was noted in all patients tested. However, plasma T_4 and T_3RU remained normal for as long as 2½ years of follow-up (Fig. 3). Administration of Sandostatin resulted in a short-term (2 h) inhibition of insulin secretion, but overall glucose

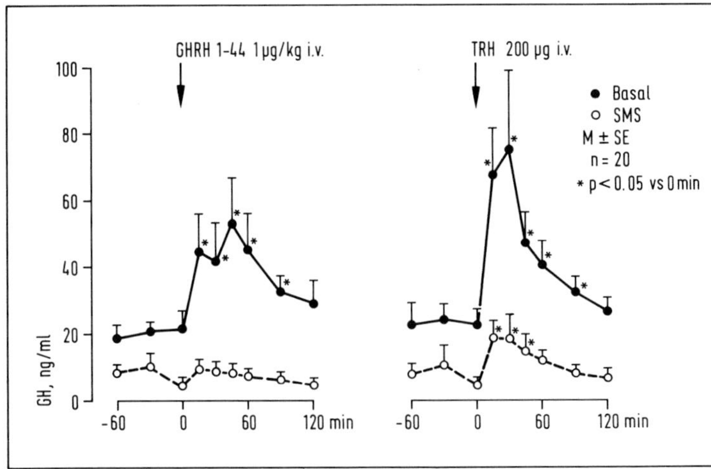

Fig. 2. Suppression of growth hormone (GH) responses to GHRH 1-44 and to TRH during Sandostatin therapy. Last injection of Sandostatin was given 60 min prior to GHRH or TRH administration. *GHRH* growth hormone releasing hormone, *TRH* thyrotropin releasing hormone

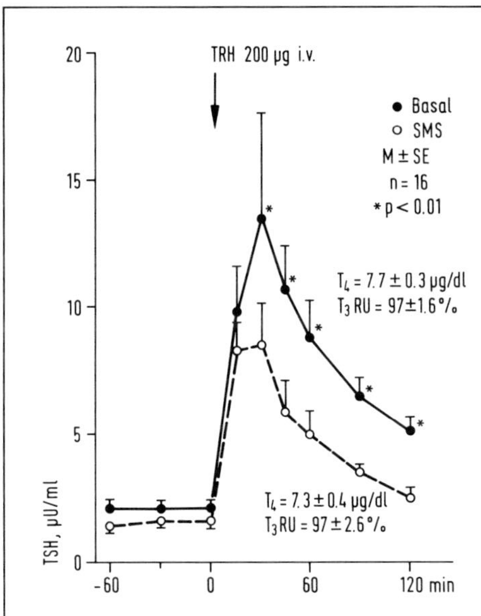

Fig. 3. Thyroid regulation before and during Sandostatin therapy in acromegalic patients. Last injection of Sandostatin was given 60 min prior to TRH administration. *TRH* thyrotropin releasing hormone, *TSH* thyroid stimulating hormone, *T₃RU* triiodothyronine resin uptake

by a normalization of plasma glucose levels throughout the day.

Pituitary Tumor Responses

In 10 previously untreated acromegalic patients, we were able to delineate the radiologic and morphologic effects of Sandostatin therapy on the tumor tissue. Significant shrinkage of the tumor was observed in all, with 20–25% shrinkage seen after 1 week of therapy, and the plateau effect (approximately 50% shrinkage) achieved after 2–3 months. This was accompanied by the diminution or frank disappearance of suprasellar and lateral extension (Fig. 4). Morphologically, Sandostatin-treated tumors were characterized by an enhanced granularity, shrinkage of total cell, nuclear and cytoplasmic volumes. Perivascular fibrosis of the tumor tissue was uniformly present, but no gross changes in tumor consistency were detected during the operation (Fig. 5).

Ectopic GHRH Secretion Syndrome

Prior to Sandostatin therapy, the patient's condition had deteriorated steadily, and liver function tests became abnormal. Pituitary hyperplasia resulted in a severe restriction of visual fields. Oncological diagnosis was that of a chemotherapy-unresponsive tumor, with a prognosis of death of the patient likely to occur within the next 6–12 months. Administration of Sandostatin,

tolerance did not change with the exception of one patient, who experienced decreased glucose tolerance (maximal plasma glucose 300 vs. 160 mg/dl before therapy). However, in another patient with frank NIDDM, Sandostatin therapy was followed

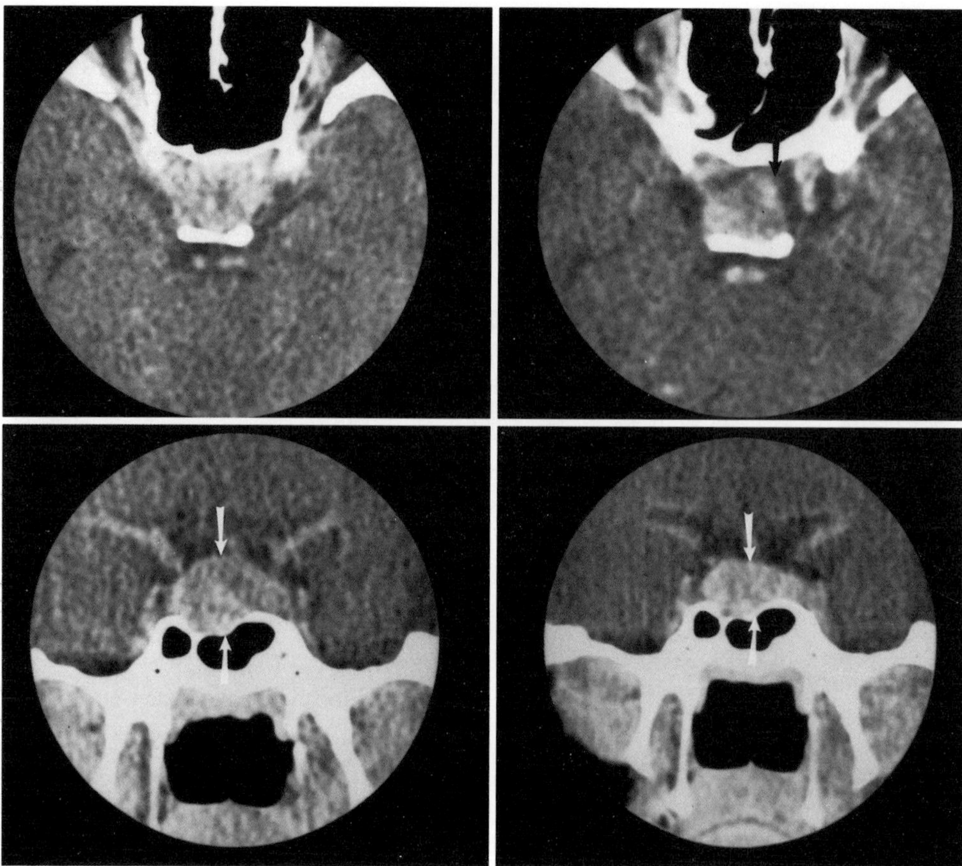

Fig. 4. Shrinkage of GH (growth hormone)-producing pituitary tumor during Sandostatin therapy

50 μg every 8 h, suppressed plasma GH and Sm-C levels to normal, and a significant shrinkage of pituitary hyperplasia with almost complete normalization of visual fields was observed. An increase in Sandostatin dose to 250 μg every 6 h was needed to suppress plasma GHRH-LI from 3.3 ± 0.6 to 1.2 ± 0.2 ng/ml. This was accompanied by a normalization of liver function and by a dramatic shrinkage of liver metastases (as judged by the abdominal CT scan). After 3 years of therapy, the patient is alive and well. He is a full-time student in a major university, actively participates in sports activities (weightlifting, riding a bicycle 20–30 mi/day), and regards himself as healthy.

Side Effects

Practically all patients noticed burning pain at the subcutaneous injection site lasting for 1–5 min. This was easily corrected by injecting the drug slowly. In approximately 50% of the patients, initiation of Sandostatin therapy was associated with abdominal cramps (10–30 min after each injection) and bloating, and in some, loose and light-colored stools also appeared. Administration of pancreatic enzymes (Viokase®) promptly relieved these symptoms. Interestingly, these complaints disappeared completely after 2–3 weeks of Sandostatin therapy and replacement enzyme treatment was not needed afterwards. In one patient, the first 2 injections of Sandostatin 250 μg were followed by nausea and severe vomiting. The decrease of the dose to 125 μg every

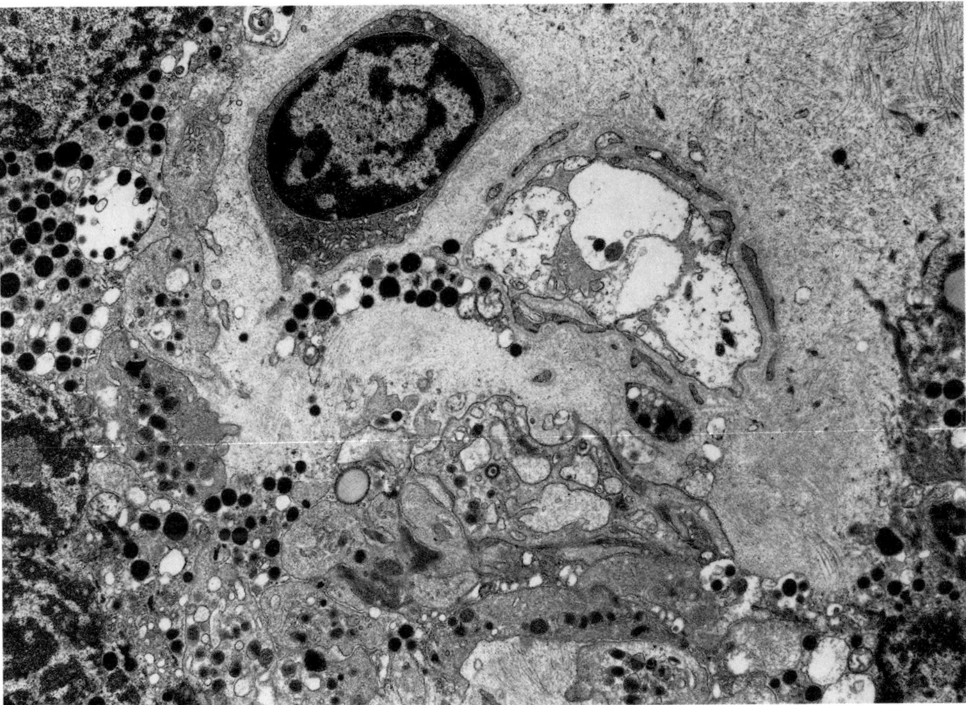

Fig. 5. Electron micrograph of a densely granulated GH (growth hormone)-producing adenoma from a patient treated with Sandostatin 50 µg q8 h for 30 weeks. There is a marked perivascular fibrosis. (x 6880)

6 h relieved these symptoms. All patients remained in the study, and all felt that clinical benefits of this therapy greatly outweighed the inconvenience of 3−4 daily injections.

Discussion

Our experience confirms the remarkable effectiveness of Sandostatin as a new pharmacologic agent for treatment of acromegaly. The better than 90% effectiveness of this drug in suppressing GH and Sm-C concentrations in patients with this disease is unequaled by any other available therapeutic modality. Furthermore, Sandostatin therapy is associated with a remarkably low incidence of serious side effects. Thus, this drug should be considered in any acromegalic patient who still has active disease postoperatively and in whom bromocriptine therapy is ineffective or cannot be tolerated. Blood glucose values should be monitored, and it may be prudent to advise

the patient to space Sandostatin injection and major meals by at least 2 h. Some patients, however, seem to be unresponsive to the GH-lowering effect of Sandostatin. This may be related to the altered number of somatostatin receptors in some GH-producing tumors [7]. However, treatment with Sandostatin may be synergistic or potentiating the effect of bromocriptine, so that a combination of both drugs may have a therapeutic effect [4].

In contrast to bromocriptine, Sandostatin has a reliable suppressive effect on GH-producing tumor growth. This is evident by the rapid shrinkage of somatotroph adenomas in Sandostatin-treated patients. This effect does not seem to be accompanied by the development of gross fibrotic changes in the tumor tissue, so that no adverse effects on the subsequent surgical results [6] are to be expected. This effect is seen also in pituitary hyperplasia owing to ectopic GHRH secretion and may be due to the abolition of the mitogenic effect of GHRH [3]. The ultimate value of the preoperative tumor shrinkage on subsequent surgical outcome remains to be determined. Additionally, Sandostatin has the ability to suppress ectopic GHRH secretion and possesses an antineoplastic effect upon GHRH-producing carcinoid tumors. The mechanism of this effect remains uncertain, but may be related to the suppression of the autocrine or paracrine growth factors [5].

Thus, Sandostatin is a remarkably effective drug for the treatment of acromegaly due to either pituitary somatotroph adenomas or ectopic GHRH secretion. It is suitable both for the long-term control of GH secretion in patients after unsuccessful surgery as well as in newly-diagnosed cases. Whether preoperative shrinkage of GH-producing macroadenomas results in a better surgical outcome needs to be confirmed.

References

1. Barkan AL, Kelch RP, Hopwood NJ, Beitins IZ (1988) Treatment of acromegaly with the long-acting somatostatin analogue SMS 201-995. J Clin Endocrinol Metab 66:16

2. Barkan AL, Shenker Y, Grekin RJ, Vale WW (1988) Acromegaly due to ectopic GHRH secretion by malignant carcinoid tumor: successful treatment with long-acting somatostatin analogue SMS 201-995. Cancer 61:221

3. Billestrup N, Swanson LW, Vale WW (1986) Growth hormone-releasing factor stimulates proliferation of somatotrophs in vitro. Proc Natl Acad Sci USA 83:6854

4. Chiodini PG, Cozzi R, Dallabonzana D, Opizzi G, Verde G, Petroncini M, Liuzzi A, Del Pozo E (1987) Medical treatment of acromegaly with SMS 201-995, a somatostatin analogue: a comparison with bromocriptine. J Clin Endocrinol Metab 64:447

5. Cuttitta F, Carney DN, Mulshine J, Moody TW, Fedorko J, Fischler A, Minna JD (1985) Bombesin-line peptides can function as autocrine growth factors in human small-cell lung cancer. Nature 316:823

6. Landolt AM, Keller PJ, Froesch ER, Mueller J (1982) Bromocriptine: does it jeopardize the result of later surgery for prolactinomas? Lancet II:657

7. Reubi JC, Heitz PU, Landolt AM (1987) Visualization of somatostatin receptors and correlation with immunoreactive growth hormone and prolactin in human pituitary adenomas: evidence for different tumor subclasses. J Clin Endocrinol Metab 65:65

15. Long-Term Treatment of Acromegaly by Continuous Subcutaneous Infusion of the Long-Acting Somatostatin Analog Sandostatin® (SMS 201-995, Octreotide)

J. P. Tauber[1], Th. Babin[1], M. C. R. Ducasse[1], M. T. Tauber[1], A. G. Harris[2], F. Bayard[1]

[1] Department of Endocrinology, Centre Hospitalier Universitaire Rangueil, Toulouse, France,
[2] Clinical Research, Sandoz Ltd, Basle, Switzerland

Recently the long-acting somatostatin analog Sandostatin® (SMS 201-995, Octreotide) was introduced for the therapy of acromegaly. On a two or three daily subcutaneous (s.c.) injection regimen plasma GH levels have been reported to be markedly decreased for several hours after each injection but tended to increase again after 6 to 8 h [3]. In order to achieve better GH control we decided to use continuous subcutaneous infusion (CSI) by means of a portable pump.

Material and Methods

Patients (Table 1)

Twelve acromegalic patients (7 men and 5 women), mean age = 43.6 years (range 18 to 74 years), were treated for a mean duration of 11.5 ± 7.3 months (range 1 to 24 months) amounting to a total drug exposure of 132 patient-months. Nine patients (5 men and 4 women) received Sandostatin as primary therapy. Four patients had a macroadenoma (grade IV), three patients had an intrasellar adenoma, and two other patients presented a normal sella turcica. Three patients (2 men and 1 woman) had previously undergone surgery (n = 3) and radiotherapy (n = 2). These three patients showed an empty sella. Growth hormone releasing hormone plasma levels were measured in all patients and found to be <30 pg/ml.

Treatment Protocol, Hormonal and Drug Measurements

Sandostatin was administered by means of a portable AS6 MP pump (Travenol, Hooksett, USA); the injection site was changed

Table 1. Characteristics of the 12 acromegalic patients

Patient	Sex	Age (years)	Previous treatment (1)	Tumoral volume (2)	$\overline{\text{m}}$GH (µg/l)	Drug treatment (3)	Duration of treatment (months)
1	F	18	0	grade IV	50.0	SMS	24
2	M	27	0	grade IV	29.4	SMS + Br	18
3	M	35	S	E	13.4	SMS	18
4	M	66	S + R	E	15.9	SMS	18
5	F	65	S + R	E	24.6	SMS	14
6	F	62	0	grade II	18.7	SMS	12
7	F	18	0	grade II	32.4	SMS	3
8	F	66	0	grade II	3.7	SMS	12
9	M	32	0	grade IV	45.7	SMS + Br	1
10	M	74	0	N	27.5	SMS	4
11	M	27	0	grade IV	8.8	SMS + Br	4
12	M	34	0	N	10.6	SMS	4

(1) 0: None, S: Surgery, R: Radiotherapy; (2) N: Normal sella turcica, E: Empty sella turcica; (3) SMS: SMS 201-995 (Sandostatin), Br: Bromocriptine

every three days and the catheter every six days. The therapeutic dose was modified monthly according to its effect on $\overline{m}GH$ (mean of 2 hourly GH determinations over 24 h) levels.

The following evaluations were carried out monthly:

GH levels were measured every two hours for 24 h at the current therapeutic dose and at a higher or a lower dose according to the results from the previous GH assessment performed one month before in order to define the lowest effective dose. GH was measured by RIA (CEA, Saclay, France).

Somatomedin-C (Sm-C) serum levels were measured by RIA according to Chatelain et al. [1]; iodinated Sm-C was purchased from Amersham (Bucks, UK). The Sm-C polyclonal antibody was kindly provided by P. Chatelain.

Sandostatin plasma levels were measured by RIA (Sandoz, Basle).

Tests of the various pituitary functions, assessments of tolerance and CT scans of the pituitary (CGR 10 000 Total Body Unit) were performed every six months by methods previously described [2].

Results

Comparative Efficacy of CSI and Multiple Injections of Sandostatin on GH Secretion (Table 2)

In three patients, plasma GH levels were compared on an identical daily dose of Sandostatin administered either by CSI or by two s.c. (8 am, 8 pm) injections. Sandostatin given twice daily did not normalize GH secretion throughout the day; complete continuous control of GH secretion could only be obtained by CSI of Sandostatin.

In three other patients, we measured plasma levels of Sandostatin on the same daily dose of Sandostatin administered by the two different methods, CSI or three s.c. injections at 8 am, 4 pm and 12 pm. Results are shown in Figure 1 for one of these patients. With CSI of 400 µg/d the plasma levels of Sandostatin ranged from 3.7 to 8.5 µg/l. Except at 8 and 10 am, the GH concentrations were lower than 5 µg/l, with a $\overline{m}GH$ of 3.6 µg/l. When the serum drug concentrations, measured after single doses, were plotted on a semilog graph as a function of time, the half-life was approximately 120 min.

Considering the values of $\overline{m}GH$ and the number of peaks >5 µg/l to assess GH secretion, three groups of patients could be defined.

Table 2

	Patient N° 3	Patient N° 4	Patient N° 6
Daily dose			
CSI	100 µg	200 µg	100 µg
MI	50 µg × 2	100 µg × 2	50 µg × 2
Results			
$\overline{m}GH$ (µg/l)			
CSI	2.1	0.7	1.4
MI	3.9	21.7	4.1
n			
CSI	0	0	0
MI	3	6	3

$\overline{m}GH$: Mean plasma GH levels as assessed from the samples taken every two hours for 24 h
n: Number of plasma GH levels >5 µg/l
CSI: Continuous subcutaneous infusion
MI: Multiple injections

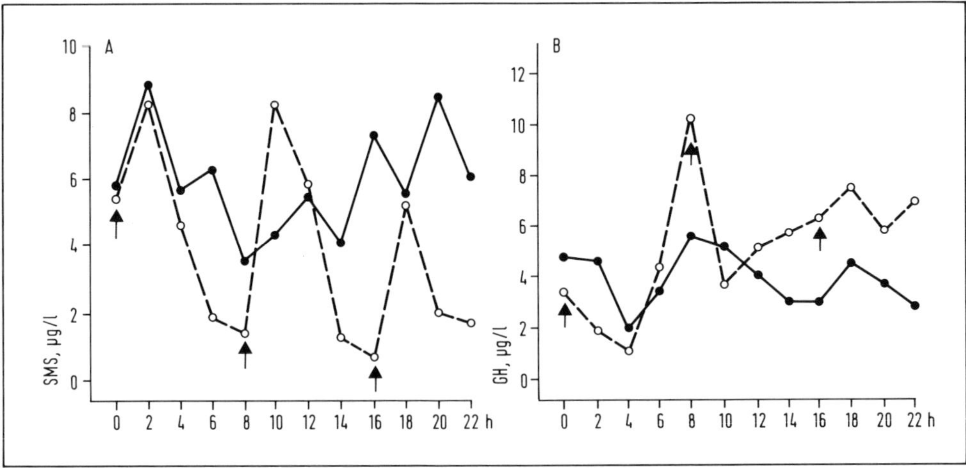

Fig. 1. Comparison of Sandostatin (SMS) (A) and GH (B) levels during continuous subcutaneous infusion at a dose of 400 µg/24 h (●——●) and during 24-h treatment by three 135 µg injections of Sandostatin (○––––○)

Group 1: 7 patients (patients 1, 3, 4, 6, 8, 10, 12) were considered well controlled (m̄GH <5 µg/l and no peak above 5 µg/l).

The initial mean dose of Sandostatin was 285 µg/d (200–600). Three patients were first treated with 200 µg/d and their daily dose had to be increased to 400 or 600 µg/d in order to achieve optimal control of GH secretion. In contrast, two patients initially treated with 400 and 600 µg/d were, later on, well controlled with 200 and 100 µg/d, respectively, and two patients initially treated with 200 µg/d are at present well controlled by 100 µg/d.

Group 2: In 4 patients (patients 2, 5, 9, 11), plasma GH levels decreased, but m̄GH remained >5 µg/l. Three patients from this incompletely controlled group also had hyperprolactinemia (patients 2, 9, 11) which was not influenced by Sandostatin. Bromocriptine (15 mg/d) was required to normalize plasma prolactin levels. Reduction of m̄GH level was gradually achieved by increasing the Sandostatin dose from a mean of 500 µg/d initially (200–600) to a mean of 1200 µg/d (800–1600).

Group 3: One patient (patient 7) was completely unresponsive to Sandostatin treatment with unmodified plasma levels of GH. Moreover the volume of the macroadenoma increased and surgery was performed after three months of Sandostatin.

After 2 to 4 weeks the patients in groups 1 and 2 showed improvement in soft tissue swelling, paresthesia, headache, asthenia, excessive sweating, and vitality.

Change in Pituitary Tumor Volume

Seven patients showed a pituitary adenoma. Three patients had an intrasellar adenoma. Two remained unchanged despite perfect control of plasma GH levels. In one patient (patient 7) the size of the adenoma increased after 3 months and surgery was performed. Four patients had a suprasellar extending macroadenoma. In one patient (patient 9) no change in pituitary tumor volume was noted after 1 month. Surgery was also performed. In three patients the size of the adenoma decreased (patients 1, 2, 11). One of these patients eventually developed an empty sella turcica after 16 months of Sandostatin therapy (patient 1).

Change in Serum Levels of Sm-C

Mean Sm-C serum level in 5 patients from group 1 decreased from 6.4 ± 3.4 U/ml to 1.7 ± 1.2 U/ml on Sandostatin treatment after 4 to 20 months. In 3 patients from the incompletely controlled group (group 2) mean Sm-C serum level decreased from 9.2 ± 2.6 U/ml before to 5.4 ± 0.6 U/ml after one to twelve months of Sandostatin.

The Sm-C serum level of the patient totally unresponsive to Sandostatin remained unchanged during the 3 months of treatment (5 U/ml).

Clinical and Biological Tolerability

Clinical tolerability was excellent, except for minor digestive problems (nausea and diarrhea) during the early days of treatment that did not appear to be dose-related. A transient rise in HbA1C levels which subsequently returned to normal within 6 to 8 months was noted. No other biological abnormality was observed. The other anterior pituitary functions were not affected by Sandostatin.

Discussion and Conclusions

Twelve acromegalic patients have been treated with Sandostatin administered by CSI with a portable pump. Despite a much longer half-life of Sandostatin compared with natural somatostatin, we confirmed the observations made by others that Sandostatin given two and even three times daily does not normalize GH secretion throughout the day in all patients. In contrast, CSI treatment with Sandostatin resulted in stable and effective Sandostatin serum levels with normalization of GH secretion, namely $\overline{m}GH < 5$ $\mu g/l$ and maximum GH peaks below 5 $\mu g/l$ over a 24-h period (12 samples). Using such criteria, therapy with Sandostatin resulted in effective control of GH hypersecretion in seven out of 12 patients with doses ranging from 100 to 600 $\mu g/d$. In four patients, receiving 800 to 1600 $\mu g/d$, partial control was obtained. Treatment with doses up to 3000 $\mu g/d$ was unsuccessful in one patient.

As also reported by others, the clinical improvement reported by the patients does not always correlate well with circulating GH and Sm-C levels [4]. In contrast, Sm-C serum levels were found to better reflect the efficacy of Sandostatin treatment on GH secretion, suggesting that efficacy of Sandostatin treatment can be evaluated by Sm-C levels combined with computerized tomography. Out of the 7 patients with a pituitary adenoma, three experienced tumor shrinkage ranging from 80% in one patient on Sandostatin treatment alone, to 25% in the two others on Sandostatin and bromocriptine; there was no change in three and an increase in one. In two patients Sandostatin was discontinued and surgery with subsequent radiotherapy was performed.

Unresponsiveness and variability in patient response both in terms of GH secretion and tumor size may be related to the density of somatostatin receptors in the pituitary.

These results demonstrate that CSI of Sandostatin achieves better and more sustained GH control than repeated s.c. injections. Moreover CSI administration of the analog may produce a more marked reduction in pituitary tumor size in some patients.

References

1. Chatelain P, van Wyk JJ, Copeland KC, Blethen SL, Underwood LE (1983) J Clin Endocrinol Metab 56:376–383
2. Ducasse MCR, Tauber JP, Tourre A, Bonafe A, Babin Th, Tauber MT, Harris AG, Bayard F (1987) J Clin Endocrinol Metab 65: 1042–1046
3. Lamberts SWJ, Oosterom R, Neufeld M, et al. (1985) J Clin Endocrinol Metab 60: 1161–1165
4. Lamberts SWJ, Uitterlinden P, Verleun T (1987) Eur J Clin Invest 17:354–359

16. Sandostatin® (SMS 201-995) Treatment of Acromegaly: Acute and Chronic Effects

S. R. George

Department of Medicine, Toronto General Hospital, University of Toronto, Toronto, Ontario, Canada

Since the present treatment of acromegaly is not optimal in normalizing growth hormone (GH) concentrations, the morbidity of the disease continues in many patients, even though they have been subjected to neurosurgery, radiotherapy and pharmacological manipulations. The effects of somatostatin [2] in inhibiting GH secretion in normal and acromegalic subjects has long been known [5, 6], yet its therapeutic potential has been limited by its short half-life and other biological effects. Since the availability of stable somatostatin analogues, there is renewed interest in this modality as a treatment for acromegaly.

The present study reports the acute and chronic effects of the somatostatin analogue SMS 201-995 (Sandostatin®) [1] in acromegalic patients.

Methods

Patients between the ages of 18 and 74 were studied. The diagnosis in each case was made on the basis of clinical features (acromegaly or gigantism), failure of GH suppression in response to an oral glucose load and the demonstration of a pituitary tumor. All but 3 of the patients had received some form of other therapy, including surgery, radiation and bromocriptine. Only one patient was an insulin-dependent diabetic. None had any known impairment of hepatic, renal, cardiovascular or circulatory function.

The acute study protocols were approved by the Human Research Ethics Committee of the Toronto General Hospital and were conducted in compliance with the principles of the Declaration of Helsinki. All patients gave informed consent. For the long-term therapeutic trials, individual approval was obtained from the Canadian Health Protection Branch, Ottawa.

Blood was sampled through an indwelling venous cannula fitted with a 3-way stopcock. On study days, subjects received standardized timed test meals.

All hormones were measured by specific radioimmunoassays, as previously described [3].

Results

The GH responses of each patient on each day were normalized about the initial fasting value. The relative changes in GH following placebo or 50 µg Sandostatin are shown in Figure 1. There was a prompt reduction in GH following administration of Sandostatin that lasted at least 6 h and rose slowly thereafter over many hours to placebo values. No rebound increase of GH was seen. In 8 of 9 patients tested thus, GH values fell to below 2 µg/l for varying lengths of time.

Profound effects were also documented on plasma insulin and C-peptide concentration. The insulin response to a meal was markedly attenuated in a dose-responsive manner by Sandostatin. The concomitant reduction of C-peptide concentrations suggested the inhibition of insulin secretion, rather than augmentation of clearance. Plasma glucose concentrations rose to diabetic values in the postprandial state.

Much less significant effects were observed on inhibition of the glucagon response. The sensitivity of effect and the duration of action of two-fold different doses of Sandostatin on inhibition of plasma GH, insulin and glucagon are shown in Figure 2.

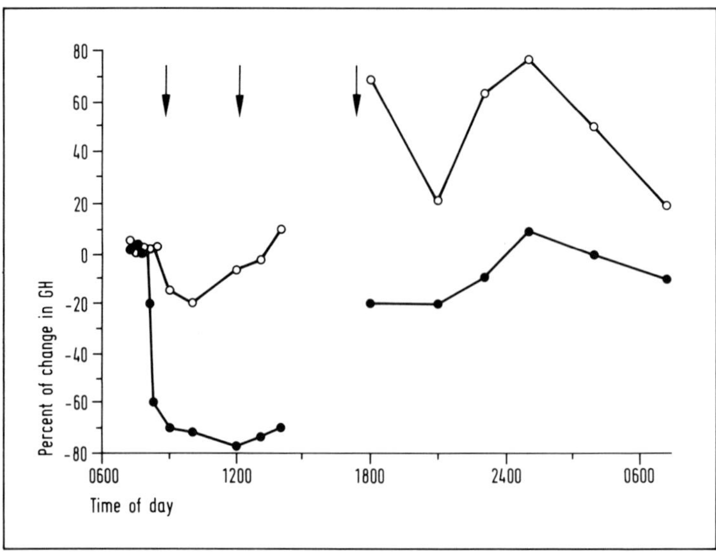

Fig. 1. Effect on growth hormone levels. ○ placebo, ● SMS (↓)

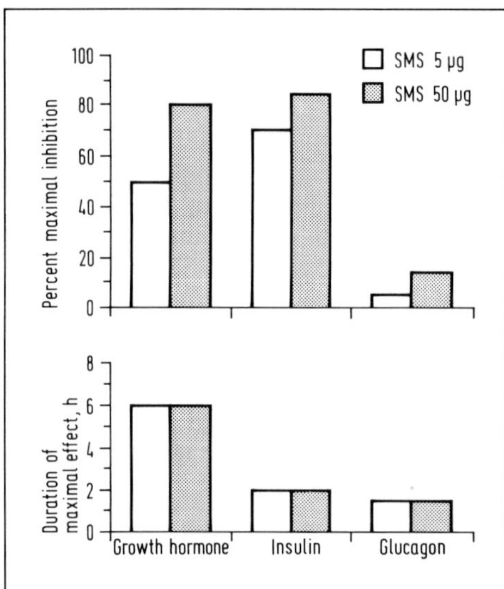

Fig. 2. Sensitivity and duration of action of Sandostatin

In each acromegalic patient, the individual duration of action and the sensitivity of effect upon GH inhibition was determined, and they were placed on q12-hourly or q8-hourly doses of Sandostatin to obtain round-the-clock inhibition of GH. In the initial part of the study, patients were maintained on this regimen for approximately 2 weeks and continued excellent GH suppression was observed. In several patients, after 1–2 weeks of Sandostatin treatment, marked improvement and normalization of OGTT was observed. Although most patients noted subjective improvement in their general well-being and level of energy, no objective changes in their nerve conduction velocities or heel-pad thickness were evident. Somatomedin-C values were lowered, but normalized only in a few.

Longer periods of treatment up to 2 years have been continued in 6 other acromegalic patients. All but 1 have had good continued suppression of GH and normalization of somatomedin-C values and glucose tolerance. The 3 longest-treated patients have had reductions in the thickness of their heel-pad. One patient has had marked reduction of suprasellar extension of tumor as documented by MR scan. One asymptomatic and two symptomatic patients have had improvement in motor and sensory nerve conduction velocities.

One patient had high GH and somatomedin-C values extremely resistant to suppression by Sandostatin even when administered by subcutaneous infusion pump. His diabetes mellitus was significantly worsened and necessitated insulin therapy. The growth of his tumor and his physical symptoms have been progressive and he is scheduled for a third neurosurgical procedure.

In a previously untreated acromegalic patient, we have documented the effects of preoperative Sandostatin treatment and found morphological changes consistent with suppression of GH release, with no evidence of cytotoxicity or vascular impairment [4].

Discussion

The present study has documented potent inhibition of GH secretion in acromegalic patients, many of whom had GH concentrations that proved resistant to normalization by other manoeuvres. The effect on pancreatic hormones, although potent, was short-lived. The far greater effect of Sandostatin on GH was well sustained and maintained as long as treatment was continued, with no evidence of desensitization or 'escape'. The metabolic consequences of GH hypersecretion also responded well to continued treatment by Sandostatin, with normalization of abnormal glucose tolerance and somatomedin-C values, reduction of soft tissue enlargement and improvement of nerve conduction parameters. Reduction of tumor size was observed only rarely. GH secretion by a very aggressive tumor in a patient could not be inhibited by the analogue. Morphological observations on a treated tumor revealed no cytotoxicity, only inhibition of hormone release, and is in agreement with the clinical observations.

In summary, Sandostatin provides a potent and well-tolerated therapeutic modality to control GH hypersecretion in acromegaly, and appears promising as first-line therapy or as an adjunct to surgical measures.

Acknowledgements: I am grateful to Sandoz (Canada and Basle) for their generous financial support of these studies, and the staff of the Clinical Investigation Unit of the Toronto General Hospital for assistance in carrying them out.

References

1. Bauer W, Briner U, Doepfner W et al. (1982) SMS 201-995: a very potent and selective octapeptide analogue of somatostatin with prolonged action. Life Sci 31:1133−1140
2. Brazeau P, Vale W, Burgus R et al. (1973) Hypothalamic peptide that inhibits the secretion of immunoreactive pituitary growth hormone. Science 179:77−79
3. George SR, Hegele RA, Burrow GN (1987) The somatostatin analogue SMS 201-995 in acromegaly: Prolonged, preferential suppression of growth hormone but not pancreatic hormones. Clin Invest Med 10:309−315
4. George SR, Kovacs K, Asa SL et al. (1987) Effect of SMS 201-995, a long-acting somatostatin analogue, on the secretion and morphology of a pituitary growth hormone cell adenoma. Clin Endocrinol 26:395−405
5. Hall R, Schally A, Evered D et al. (1973) Action of growth hormone-release inhibitory hormones in healthy men and in acromegaly. Lancet II:581−584
6. Yen S, Siler T, Devane G (1974) Effect of somatostatin in patients with acromegaly. N Engl J Med 290:935−938

17. Long-Term Efficacy of Sandostatin® (SMS 201-995, Octreotide) in 178 Acromegalic Patients. Results from the International Multicentre Acromegaly Study Group*

A. G. Harris, H. Prestele, K. Herold, V. Boerlin

Department Neuroendocrinology and Biostatistics, Clinical Research, Sandoz Ltd, Basle, Switzerland

Sandostatin® (SMS 201-995), a synthetic long-acting octapeptide, represents an efficacious alternative therapeutic candidate to available treatment modalities for acromegaly.

Indeed, the principle actions of Sandostatin on the pituitary are its ability to inhibit, in normal subjects, exercise-stimulated growth hormone (GH) secretion, arginine-stimulated GH secretion, sleep-induced GH secretion, release of GH by insulin-induced hypoglycemia, TRH-stimulated release of TSH, postprandial release of insulin, glucagon, gastrin and other peptides of the gastroenteropancreatic system.

The first report by Plewe et al. [8] showed that 50 µg Sandostatin s.c. could reduce GH levels to below 2 ng/ml for up to 9 h in 6 out of 7 acromegalic patients without any rebound phenomenon or undue side effects. Subsequently, compassionate-need acromegalic patients as well as a limited number of trial subjects were treated with Sandostatin and are the subject of this report.

Patients and Methods

Collectively, 178 patients (78 males and 100 females) with active acromegaly were treated at 22 centres. 135 patients had been previously treated (surgery, radiation, bromocriptine) and the remaining 43 were untreated. Patients' ages ranged from 18 to 77 years (median 49 years). Patients were to have clinically active acromegaly, confirmed by the presence of mean elevated basal levels of GH above 5 ng/ml and/or the lack of GH suppressibility to below 2 ng/ml following a 75 or 100 g oral glucose tolerance test (OGTT) and/or increased somatomedin-C (Sm-C) levels above the upper normal limit. Recommendations for drug administration were made on the basis of individual dose titration depending on patients' clinical and biochemical response and tolerability from a starting dose of 50 µg to a final dose of 500 µg b.i.d. or t.i.d. subcutaneously. A limited number of patients were given Sandostatin by continuous subcutaneous infusion (CSI).

The most frequently observed clinical signs and symptoms reported were: excessive sweating in 137 patients, acral features in 174, and soft tissue swelling in 172. Measurements of hand size (ring size or hand volume) were made in 40 patients.

* Clinical Investigators: R. Astorga/P. P. Garcia-Luna/A. Leal del Cerro (Sevilla, Spain); S. Boyages/ C. Eastman/H. Smith (NSW, Aus); W. Burr (Wakefield, G.B.); B. Glaser (Jerusalem, IL); S. George/ G. N. Burrow (Toronto, CDN); G. Pieters, P. A. van Liessum (Nijmegen, NL); E. F. Pfeiffer/L. Duntas (Ulm, D); J. Pichel (Erlangen, D); K. Ho/L. Lazarus (Sydney, Aus); E. Vilardell (Barcelona, Spain); G. Tolis (Athens, GR); F. Bayard/J. P. Tauber/Th. Babin (Toulouse, F); R. A. Donald (Christchurch, NZ); G. M. Besser/W. Wass (London, G.B.); R. Hall/M. Scanlon (Cardiff, G.B.); S. W. J. Lamberts (Rotterdam, NL); J. Lubetzki/Ph. Chanson/J. Timsit/A. Warnet (Paris, F); A. Beckers/A. Stevenaert/G. Hennen (Liège, B); G. Pagani/M. Salmoiraghi (Bergamo, I); H. J. Quabbe/U. Plöckinger (Berlin, D); H. Ørskov/J. Weeke/S. E. Christensen (Aarhus, DK); R. A. Liuzzi/P. G. Chiodini/R. Cozzi (Milano, I).
Coordination: A. G. Harris
Statistical Evaluation: H. Prestele
Data Processing: K. Herold, C. Frame, G. Kuntzelmann, G. Haas, J. Fischer, A. Meier-Hornig
Technical Assistance: R. Hasemer, J. Millar, A. Albitz

Mean and median Sandostatin dosage were 253 µg and 200 µg/day respectively. Range of dosage was 50–1500 µg/day. The doses most commonly administered were 100 µg s.c., b.i.d. and t.i.d. in 50 and 64 patients respectively. Total drug exposure amounted to 40 149 patient-days.

CT scans of the pituitary fossa and neighbouring structures were performed in 110 patients prior to Sandostatin therapy. In 81, a demonstrable pituitary tumour was found. Measurement of tumour mass was made in 34 patients at baseline and during Sandostatin treatment.

The main parameters of efficacy evaluated were the effect of Sandostatin on serum GH and Sm-C, as well as control of symptoms and signs and tumour size reduction.

Since the number of GH determinations were highly variable from one patient to another, only 149 (83.7%) of 178 patients from whom a minimum of six samples of serum per visit, collected over a time period of 6–24 h and assayed for GH, were statistically evaluated. Thus 8276 GH values out of 11078 were assessed.

Somatomedin-C serum levels were measured at baseline and during Sandostatin therapy in 165 patients.

The data submitted here were reviewed with the aim of establishing whether in acromegalic patients Sandostatin can:

1. reduce elevated levels of GH and Sm-C;
2. ameliorate the severity of the signs and symptoms of the disease;
3. reduce GH secretion more markedly than currently available medical therapy (dopamine agonists, e.g. bromocriptine);
4. reduce pituitary tumour size in some instances;
5. produce the clinical response with an acceptable margin of safety.

Results

Growth Hormone and Somatomedin-C Response to Sandostatin (Figs. 1 and 2)

If one accepts a GH cut-off level equal to or below 10 ng/ml, then 74.5% of the patients in this series were responders.

If one accepts GH values above 10 ng/ml but more than a 50% reduction of GH pretreatment levels, then an additional 12.8% of patients are found to be partial responders.

At the 5 ng/ml level 68 (46%) patients have 75% of their individual GH profile measurements within this limit.

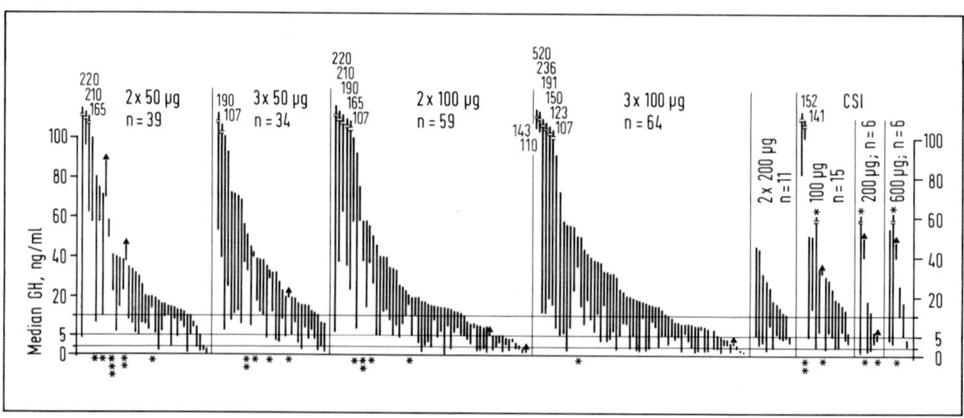

Fig. 1. Reduction of growth hormone (GH) levels. Each patient is represented by a vertical bar indicating pretreatment median GH levels and pooled median GH value on Sandostatin dose (daily dose shown in figure). * = non-responder; ↑ = increase; *CSI* continuous subcutaneous infusion

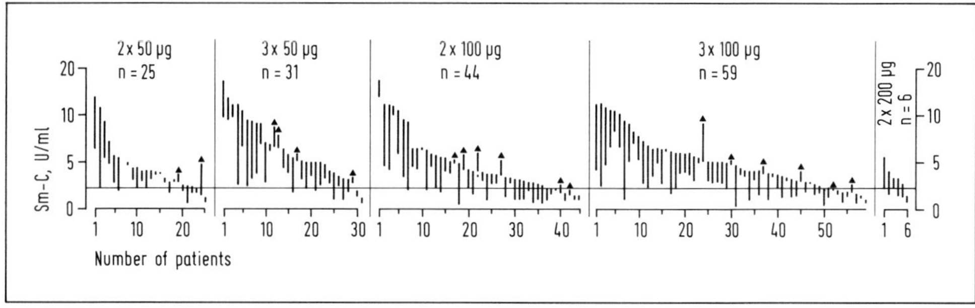

Fig. 2. Reduction in somatomedin-C (Sm-C) levels. Each patient is represented by a vertical bar indicating patient number and Sm-C levels before and during Sandostatin therapy (daily dose shown)

If normalization is defined as GH ≤2 ng/ml, 31 (20.8%) patients were normalized.

Sm-C plasma levels were reduced by 20 to 50% depending on Sandostatin dose and normalized in 61/165 (36%) patients.

Neither rebound phenomena nor tachyphylaxis have been reported in acromegalic patients treated with Sandostatin.

Symptom Improvement

Clinical symptoms were significantly improved in most patients (Fig. 3).

An outstanding feature of Sandostatin which was reported shortly after its introduction [6] is the rapid onset of clinical improvement which occurs within days.

Headache, a common finding in acromegaly was reported by 94 of the patients in this series, 84% of whom improved on Sandostatin.

Sweating was greatly reduced and soft tissue swelling was significantly diminished. Intermittent sleep apnea markedly improved in one out of 3 patients in the series who suffered from this disorder at baseline.

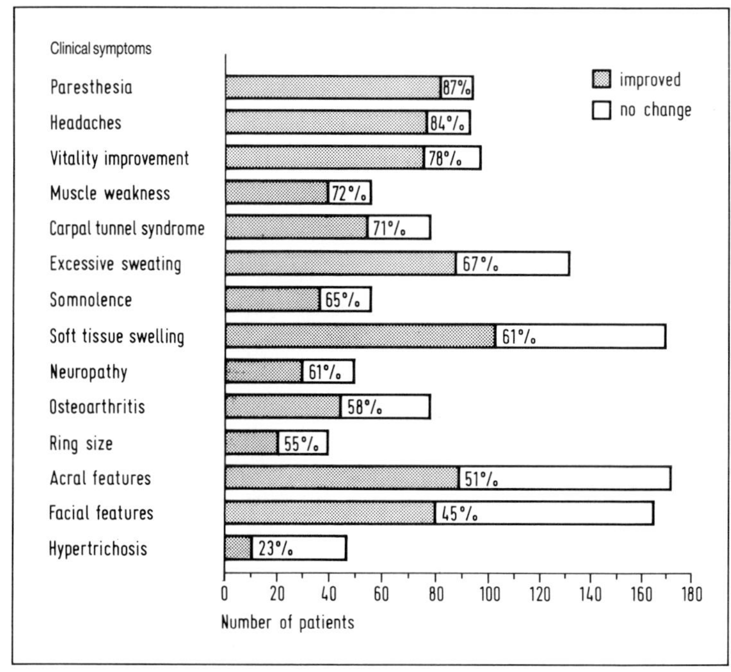

Fig. 3. Improvement in clinical symptoms. n = 175/178

Eight out of 17 patients in the present collection showed an improvement in dyspnea. One of these patients had end-stage heart failure and was scheduled to undergo heart transplantation which was avoided through Sandostatin therapy. Moreover, cardiomegaly was reduced in 2 patients.

Pituitary Tumour Shrinkage

Of 26 patients, in whom transversal diameters were measured, 8 (30.8%) had at least a 20% decrease. Nineteen of 31 patients (41.9%) showed a decrease in the vertical diameter of at least 20%. Finally, 2 of 24 (8.3%) patients had a decrease of at least 20% in the anteroposterior diameter.

Figure 4 shows tumour size reduction on magnetic resonance imaging and Figure 5 positron emission tomography during Sandostatin therapy in a 28-year-old male acromegalic who was resistant to surgery and bromocriptine.

The most marked tumour size reductions have been obtained on CSI administration of Sandostatin. An 80% pituitary tumour size reduction has been noted in 1 acromegalic patient after 600 µg/24 h Sandostatin given by CSI for 4 months. GH control and tumour shrinkage were maintained despite subsequent reduction of Sandostatin dose to 100 µg/24 h [5].

Comparative Efficacy with Bromocriptine

Published data demonstrates a faster, more powerful and more prolonged maximum GH suppression on Sandostatin compared with bromocriptine [1, 2, 4, 7, 11].

Safety and Tolerability

Adverse Events

Sandostatin was well tolerated up to 1500 µg per day over a period ranging from 6 days to 35.4 months.

Eleven patients reported effects at the site of injection. The pain experienced by them is presumably related to the acetic acid vehicle solution.

Sandostatin treatment is associated with a variety of gastrointestinal adverse effects, including nausea, vomiting, flatulence, abdominal discomfort, diarrhea and pale stools which sometimes resemble steatorrhea in appearance. In one patient, Sando-

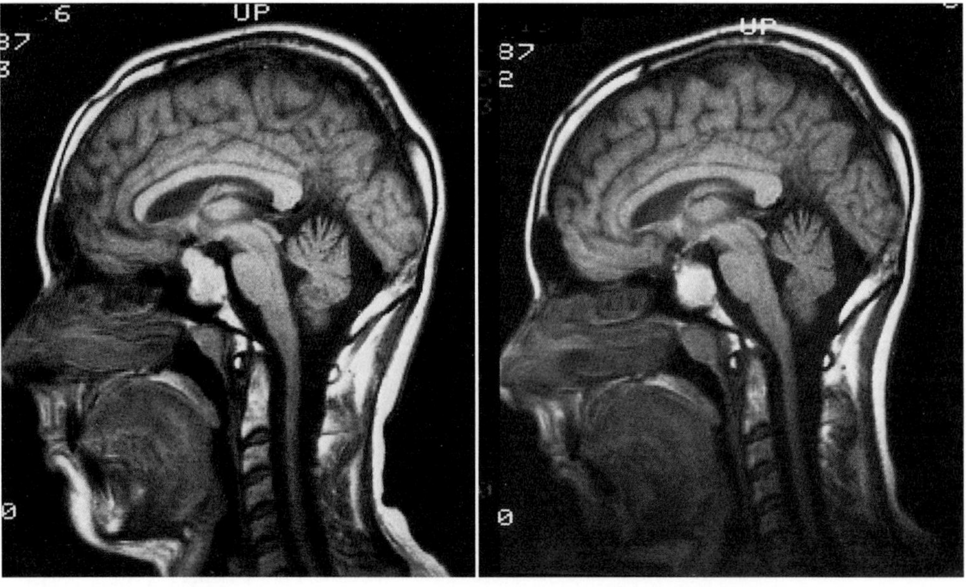

Before   400 µg Sandostatin t.i.d.

Fig. 4. Reduction in tumour size (magnetic resonance imaging). (Sorce as Fig. 5)

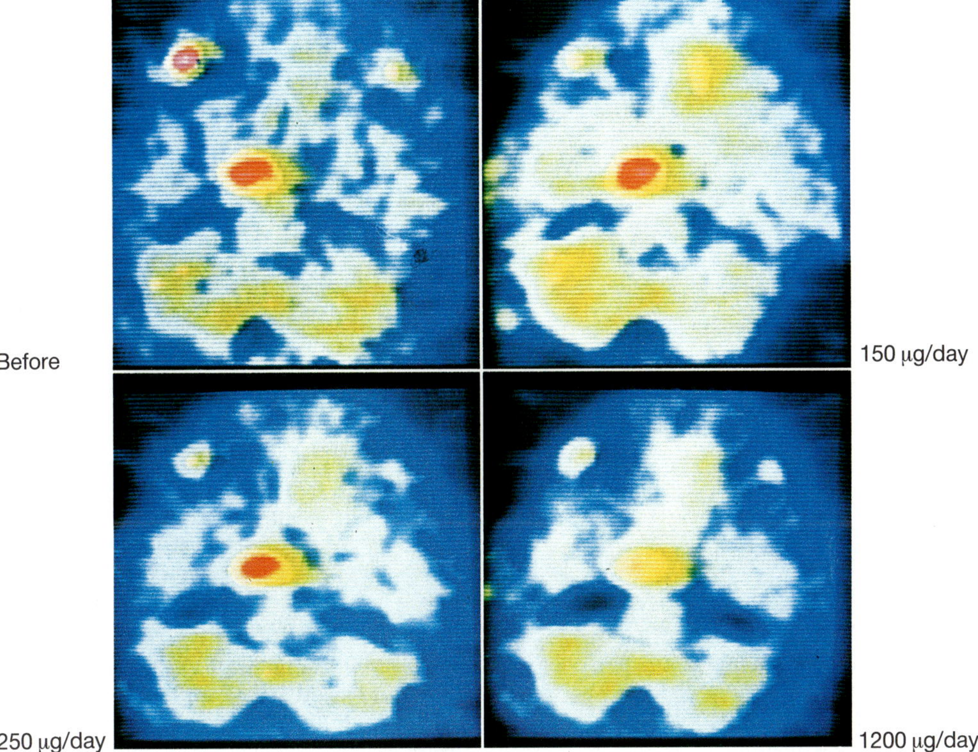

Fig. 5. Reduction in pituitary tumor size during Sandostatin therapy shown (positron emission tomography). (Pictures by courtesy of P. O. Lundberg, C. Muhr and M. Bergström, University of Uppsala, Sweden)

statin was discontinued due to the severity of the adverse effect (diarrhea).

Asymptomatic gallstones were reported in three patients.

Antibody formation to Sandostatin has not yet been reported in patients treated with the analogue.

Overall, 62 patients (34.4%) reported one or more adverse events. In most cases the event was reported spontaneously by the patient (67.4%) and most were rated as mild or moderate in severity (93.2%) (Fig. 6).

Sandostatin has had no consistent effect on the clinical chemistry or haematological parameters evaluated. Anaemia noted in some patients was due to frequent blood sampling for hormonal profiles.

Glucose Tolerance

Despite significant insulin inhibition by 20 to 50% on various Sandostatin doses, blood glucose levels increased only by 1−2 mmol/l on average. These results suggest that suppressed insulin levels are outweighed by Sandostatin's inhibitory effect on growth hormone (Fig. 7).

Thyroid Hormones

Sandostatin did not influence the basal values of TSH, T_3 or T_4.

Discussion and Conclusions

Efficacy

The primary objective of therapy should be cure of the acromegaly. Results obtained with Sandostatin in the patients included in this series should be considered in the context of alternative therapeutic options. Unfortunately, there is no agreed definition of

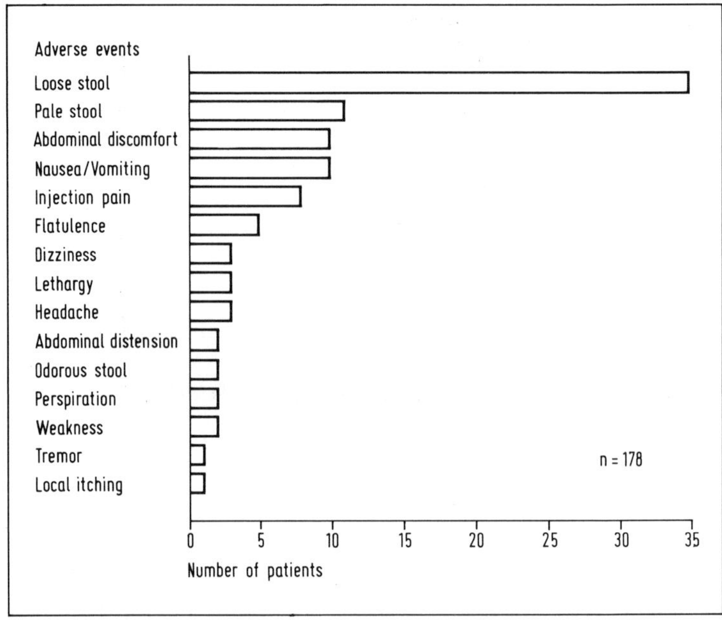

Fig. 6. Adverse effects. In addition to the side effects shown in the figure, the following were reported once each: muscle cramps, hair loss, local pain, rash at injection site, hypotension, and anorexia

cured acromegaly. Moreover, some authors use single basal GH levels whilst others perform GH profiles or measure mean GH concentration during an oral glucose load as an index of biochemical control. To date, it has been considered that "cure" (arbitrarily defined in the literature as GH <5 or <10 ng/ml) can only be achieved by transsphenoidal resection of microadenomas or moderate-sized macroadenomas. As shown in Table 1 [13], success rates vary quite dramatically from 44 to 90%, depending on the skill of the surgeon and the size of the tumour and on the criterion adopted for evaluating cure (GH <5 or <10 ng/ml). Most patients with large tumours benefit

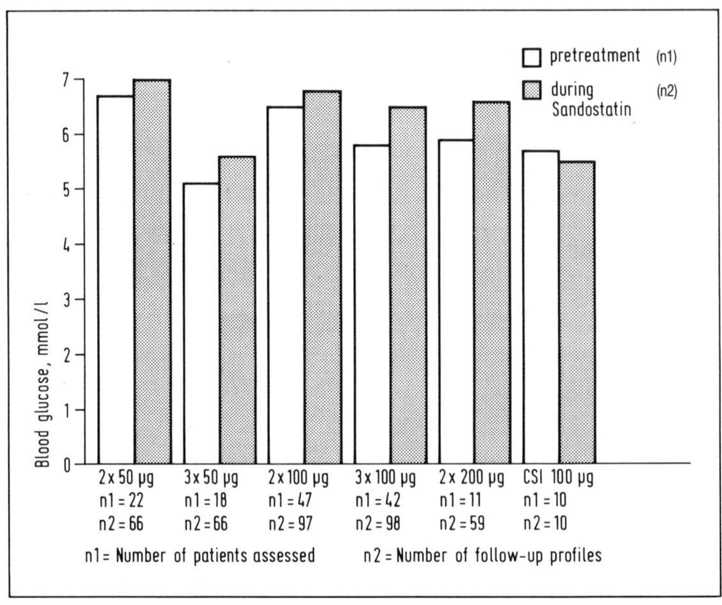

Fig. 7. Carbohydrate tolerance. (Daily dose of Sandostatin shown)

from size reduction by operation but "cure" is rarely obtained, and in such cases radiotherapy is required. However, radiotherapy usually takes 2 to 10 years to achieve normalization of GH levels and causes hypopituitarism in a significant proportion of cases. Moreover, the frequency of recurrence of the disease after surgery is still poorly known. Bromocriptine is often recommended as adjunctive therapy while awaiting the full effects of irradiation.

Radiotherapy and/or bromocriptine may be used as primary treatment in patients who are at risk for surgery or in elderly patients with only modest GH elevations.

Bromocriptine may be given alone to young patients in whom preservation of fertility is important. However, bromocriptine normalizes GH in only 20–30% of patients.

The wealth of data and the depth of critical analysis together with the criteria applied (GH profiles including no less than 6 GH determinations evaluated according to various definitions of biochemical cure), from the present series, which represents the largest single collection of acromegalic patients to date treated with a single medication, shows that Sandostatin therapy achieves a higher clinical and biochemical response rate than the current available treatment modalities. The fact that 135 out of the 178 acromegalic patients included in this submission had already failed to respond to either surgery, radiation or bromocriptine or a combination of 2 or all 3, strengthens the therapeutic claim that Sandostatin is highly effective in the treatment of acromegalic patients who have failed to respond to these modalities. Furthermore, Sandostatin should be useful:

- in the interim period until radiotherapy is fully effective;
- in young male acromegalic patients in whom preservation of fertility is important;
- in acromegalic patients unfit or unwilling to undergo surgery.

Table 1. Results of transsphenoidal surgery in acromegaly

Series	Number of cases	Number cured	Per-centage	Surgically related hypopi-tuitarism	Surgical mortality (%)	Level of GH used as criteria for cure (ng/ml)
Arafah, 1980	25	17	68	12	0	< 5
Balagura, 1981	132	–	58	*	*	< 5
Bøhmer, 1974	23	16	70	17	0	< 6
Emory series, 1985	64	45	70	8	0	< 5
Faglia, 1978	18	12	67	17	§	<10
Garcia-Uria, 1978	41	31	78	10	0	<10
Giovanelli, 1976	27	12	44	*	0	<10
Giovanelli, Fahlbusch et al., 1980	57	47	82	7	0	< 5
Hardy, 1979	120	94	78	11	0.8	< 5
Laws, 1979	80	53	66	16	0	<10
Leavens, 1977	16	12	75		0	< 5
Lüdecke, 1976	80	70	87.5	*	0	< 5
Quabbe, 1982**	152	83 (GH<5) 121 (<10)	55	17	–	< 5
Teasdale, 1982	28	19	68	25	0	<10
Tucker, 1980	32	24	75	13	0	< 5
Williams, 1975	59	39	66	*	0	< 5
Wilson et al., 1982	137	106	77	2	0	<10

* Incidence not clear from report
§ Not mentioned in report
** Multicentre report

Sandostatin may also prove to be a useful adjunct in reducing pituitary adenoma size and softening tumour tissue prior to surgery. No rebound GH hypersecretion after cessation of treatment of tachyphylaxis have been observed.

Dosage and Administration

The data from this series indicate that the maintenance dose for most patients with acromegaly is 100 µg administered subcutaneously three times daily. However, the dose range over which GH and Sm-C reduction and symptom control as well as tumour shrinkage may be obtained is 50 µg b.i.d. to 500 µg t.i.d. Doses of up to 600 µg/24 h given by CSI may be required in some patients. Progressively higher doses of Sandostatin have not led to response attenuation or to desensitization, since GH in some patients has been shown to be completely suppressed with long-term subcutaneous infusion of Sandostatin using a pump. In fact, two patients on CSI in this series were able to reduce their starting dose of 600 µg/24 h to 100 µg/24 h after 4 months with the same GH-lowering effect. In some patients CSI of Sandostatin may achieve more effective and sustained suppression of GH and Sm-C levels in acromegaly compared with repeated s.c. injections of the analogue as suggested by Cozzi et al. [3] and Timsit et al. [12].

In a series of 12 acromegalic patients given 100, 200 and 500 µg Sandostatin t.i.d. GH data showed that doses above 100 µg t.i.d. do not produce a further significant suppression of GH plasma concentrations [9].

This variation in dosage requirements may be due to the varying sensitivities of individual pituitary adenomas to Sandostatin treatment, depending on the density of somatostatin receptors in the gland [10].

The initial recommended dosage is 50–100 µg Sandostatin by subcutaneous injection every 8 or 12 h. Patients should be re-evaluated monthly and the dosage adjusted on the basis of reduction of growth hormone or clinical response. The usual optimal therapeutic dosage range of Sandostatin varies from 200 to 300 µg per day in most patients. The maximum dosage should not exceed 1500 µg per day.

If, during Sandostatin therapy, no significant reduction in growth hormone levels takes place, careful assessment of the clinical features of the disease should be made and, if no change has occurred, dosage adjustment or discontinuation of therapy should be considered.

In elderly patients treated with Sandostatin, there was no evidence for reduced tolerability or altered dosage requirements. Experience with Sandostatin in children is very limited.

Overdosage

The maximum single dose so far given to healthy volunteers has been 1000 µg by intravenous bolus injection. The observed signs and symptoms were a brief drop in heart rate, facial flushing, abdominal cramps, diarrhea, an empty feeling in the stomach and nausea which resolved within 24 h of drug administration.

No life-threatening reactions have been reported after acute overdosage. One patient has been reported to have received an accidental overdose of Sandostatin by continuous infusion (250 µg/h for 48 h instead of 25 µg/h). He experienced no side effects.

The management of overdosage is symptomatic.

References

1. Borges F, Francis D, Davidson K et al. (1987) Nocturnal secretion of growth hormone during treatment of acromegaly with somatostatin analogue and bromocriptine. J Endocrinol [Suppl 112]: Abstract 88
2. Chiodini PG, Cozzi R, Dallabonzana D et al. (1987) Medical treatment of acromegaly with SMS 201-995, a somatostatin analogue: a comparison with bromocriptine. J Clin Endocrinol 64:447–453
3. Cozzi R, Chiodini PG, Dallabonzana D et al. (1986) Infusion of somatostatin analogue SMS 201-995: a comparison with subcutaneous intermittent administration. Somatostatin Symposium, Washington, May 1986, Abstract 11–15
4. Cozzi R, Dallabonzana D, Oppizzi G, Verde G et al. (1986) Medical treatment of acromegaly with SMS 201-995, a new somatosta-

tin analogue: a comparison with bromocriptine. Neuroendocrine Perspectives 5: 161–166

5. Ducasse MCR, Tauber JP, Tourre A et al. (1987) Dramatic shrinking effect of somatostatin analogue SMS 201-995 on GH-producing pituitary tumours. J Clin Endocrinol Metab 65:1042–1046

6. Lamberts SWJ, Uitterlinden P, Verschoor L et al. (1985) Long-term treatment of acromegaly with somatostatin analogue SMS 201-995. N Engl J Med 313:1576–1585

7. Lamberts SWJ, Zweens M, Verschoor L et al. (1986) A comparison among growth hormone-lowering effects in acromegaly of the somatostatin analogue SMS 201-995, bromocriptine and the combination of both drugs. J Clin Endocrinol 63:16–19

8. Plewe G, Beyer J, Krause U et al. (1984) Long acting and selective suppression of growth hormone secretion by somatostatin analogue 201-995 in acromegaly. Lancet II:782–784

9. Plöckinger U, Quabbe HJ (1987) Treatment of acromegaly with somatostatin analogue SMS 201-995; dose-response study and long-term effectiveness. 1st European Congress of Endocrinology, Abstract 1–17

10. Reubi JC, Heitz PU, Landolt AM (1987) Visualization of somatostatin receptor and correlation with immunoreactive GH and prolactin in human pituitary adenomas: Evidence for different tumour subclasses. J Clin Endocrinol Metab 65:65–73

11. Sandler LM, Burrin JM, Williams G et al. (1987) Effective long-term treatment of acromegaly with a long-acting somatostatin analogue (SMS 201-995). Clin Endocrinol 26:85–95

12. Timsit J, Chanson P, Larger E et al. (1987) The effect of subcutaneous injections of a somatostatin analogue (SMS 201-995) on the diurnal GH profile in acromegaly. Acta Endocrinol 116:118–112

13. Tindall GT, Barrow DL (eds) (1986) Disorders of the pituitary. Mosby, St. Louis

18a. Pulsatile Administration of SMS 201-995 (Sandostatin®) in the Treatment of Acromegaly

H. Imura, Y. Kato, N. Hattori

Department of Medicine, Kyoto University, Faculty of Medicine, Kyoto, Japan, and Department of Medicine, Shimane Medical University, Izumo City, Shimane, Japan

A potent long-acting analogue of somatostatin, SMS 201-995 (Sandostatin®), has been reported to be effective in the treatment of acromegaly [2, 3]. The usual dose regimens used in these treatments were 2 to 3 subcutaneous injections per day. It has been observed, however, that such patterns of administration do not consistently lower plasma GH levels, due to a limited duration of action of this peptide. In order to achieve more consistent suppression of plasma GH and better therapeutic efficacy, we tried to give Sandostatin in a pulsatile way by using an infusion pump.

Two male and three female acromegalic patients who had elevated basal plasma GH levels were subjected to this study. All of them had previously undergone transsphenoidal adenomectomy but had elevated plasma GH levels because of residual tumors. An infusion pump (Nipro Co., Tokyo) which was originally designed for the pulsatile administration of LHRH was used in all subjects and the initial dose was 10 µg of the peptide every 2 h. The dose was increased, if necessary, and in one patient the frequency of pulse was increased from 12 to 16 times a day because of the return of headache. Plasma GH was measured by the conventional double antibody radioimmunoassay and plasma somatomedin-C (Sm-C) by the RIA kit of Nichols Institute. Urinary GH excretion was measured in 24-h pooled urine by a sandwich enzyme immunoassay [1] and expressed as ng/g creatinine.

As a preliminary experiment, 10, 15, 50 and 100 µg of Sandostatin were injected subcutaneously and plasma GH was measured serially. Plasma GH was decreased to below 20% of the basal level by the peptide at all doses used, with the nadir after 2 h. The duration of action was longer when larger amounts of the peptide were used. On the basis of these results we adopted 10 µg as the initial Sandostatin dose and 2 h as the interval of pulsatile injection.

Repeated pulsatile administration of Sandostatin significantly lowered plasma GH levels in all patients studied. Compared with the 2−3 daily injections, plasma GH levels were consistently low throughout the day, as a representative result in Figure 1 shows. The dose required was 120 to 300 µg/day except for one patient who needed larger doses. Urinary GH excretion which reflects daily GH secretory rate [1] also decreased remarkably, consistent with the observation that plasma GH remained low throughout a day. Plasma somatomedin-C levels were also decreased to the values below 2 U/ml (in all cases) after the treatment.

Clinical improvements were brought about in all patients. Decreased sweating, relieved headache and improvements of glucose tolerance curves were observed in these cases. One patient who had mild headache before the treatment complained of severe headache of rebound type a few hours after the subcutaneous injection of Sandostatin. Pulsatile administration of Sandostatin promptly relieved the headache but this returned 1.5 h later. We therefore shortened the interval of pulse from 2 h to 1.5 h and succeeded in controlling headache in this patient. Soft tissue thickness seemed also to be improved. No serious side effects were noted in the patients and there were complaints of only mild pain at the site of injection.

The suppressive effect of Sandostatin lasted even after prolonged treatment with the infusion pump and the longest period of

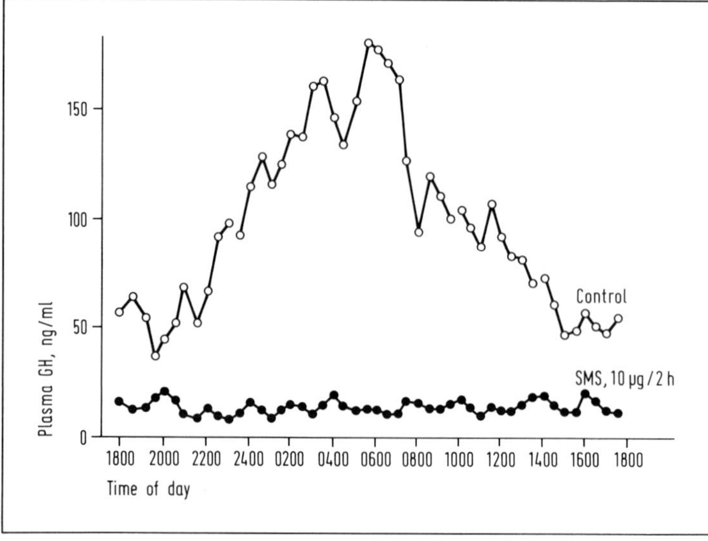

Fig. 1. Diurnal changes of plasma growth hormone (GH) in a patient with acromegaly before (open circle) and during (closed circle) the pulsatile treatment with Sandostatin using an infusion pump (10 µg SMS every 2 h)

treatment is more than one year. This indicates that pulsatile administration of Sandostatin does not induce down regulation or desensitization, even after prolonged treatment. Timsit et al. [4] reported similar results with continuous subcutaneous injection of 100 µg of Sandostatin. They did not observe any phenomenon compatible with down regulation, although their trial was of short duration.

In conclusion, pulsatile administration of Sandostatin was effective in consistently lowering plasma GH in patients who did not respond optimally to 2 to 3 times daily injection.

References

1. Hattori N, Kato Y, Murakami Y, Koshiyama H, Inoue T, Imura H (1987) Measurement of urine human growth hormone levels by ultra-highly sensitive enzyme immunoassay. Folia Endocrinol Jpn (in press)
2. Lamberts SWJ, Uitterlinden P, Verschoor L, van Dongen KJ, Del Pozo E (1985) Long-term treatment of acromegaly with the somatostatin analogue SMS 201-995. N Engl J Med 313:1576−1580
3. Plewe G, Beyer J, Krause U, Neufeld M, Del Pozo E (1984) Long-acting and selective suppression of growth hormone secretion by somatostatin analogue SMS 201-995 in acromegaly. Lancet II:782−784
4. Timsit J, Chanson P, Larger E, Duet M, Mosse A, Guillausseau PJ, Harris AG, Moulonguet M, Warnet A, Lubetzki J (1987) The effect of subcutaneous infusion versus subcutaneous injection of a somatostatin analogue (SMS 201-995) on the diurnal GH profile in acromegaly. Acta Endocrinol 116: 108−112

18b. Treatment of Acromegaly with SMS 201-995 (Sandostatin®): A Collaborative Study in Japan

H. Imura, M. Irie

Department of Medicine, Kyoto University Faculty of Medicine, Kyoto, Japan, and Department of Medicine, Toho University School of Medicine, Tokyo, Japan

Dopaminergic agonists, such as bromocriptine, have been used for the medical management of acromegaly, but their GH-suppressing effect is either incomplete or absent in a certain number of patients. More recently, SMS 201-995 (Sandostatin®), a long-acting somatostatin analogue, has become available and been reported to be effective in most of the patients with acromegaly [1, 3]. This communication describes an investigation in Japan, which was a collaborative study of several institutions.

Twenty-three acromegalic patients, 7 males and 16 females, aged 22 to 73, were selected for this study. Bromocriptine was previously used in 14 patients but was ineffective except in one patient. A single subcutaneous injection of 50 µg of Sandostatin was performed in 18 patients and plasma GH was measured up to 24 h after the injection. The therapeutic dose of Sandostatin was 50 µg, b.i.d. initially and then increased to either 50 µg, t.i.d. or 100 µg, b.i.d. if necessary. In 4 patients, the dose was further increased to 100 µg, t.i.d. For seven days plasma GH was measured every morning at resting state before the Sandostatin injection, and then once every week. A commercial kit was used for GH radioimmunoassay (RIA). Plasma somatomedin-C (Sm-C) was measured by the RIA kit of Nichols Institute before, and 1 to 11 weeks after, the beginning of treatment. Clinical manifestations and side effects were observed by doctors.

Figure 1 illustrates changes of plasma GH in response to a single subcutaneous injection of 50 µg Sandostatin in 18 acromegalic patients studied. Plasma GH decreased rapidly, reaching the nadir at 2 h and recovering gradually to pre-injection levels at 12 h. Twelve of 18 subjects were known to

be unresponsive to a single oral administration of 2.5 mg bromocriptine. This indicates that Sandostatin is effective in lowering plasma GH level in patients who are resistant to bromocriptine.

Results of repeated Sandostatin administration are shown in Figure 2. Morning levels of plasma GH decreased gradually during the treatment with Sandostatin in 15 patients and reached the levels below 5 ng/ml in 8 patients. On the other hand, plasma GH levels were virtually unchanged in the remaining 8 patients. Among the latter, the dose of Sandostatin or the frequency of subcutaneous injections was insufficient in 6 (less than 100 µg per day or 2 daily injections, respectively). The remaining two patients received 100 µg t.i.d. with no significant effect on the morning plasma GH levels. Their response to a single injection of this peptide was also relatively poor compared with responders, with the nadir value more than 50% of the pre-injection level.

Plasma Sm-C levels significantly decreased in 11 of 15 patients studied but the level below 2 U/ml was achieved in only 6 patients. Clinical symptoms such as sweating, headache, paresthesia of the extremities and a heavy sensation in the head were improved in responders. As for untoward effects, pain at the site of injection, epigastric discomfort, nausea, and diarrhea were noted in 30, 17, 9 and 4% of the patients, respectively.

Previous studies have shown that repeated subcutaneous injection of Sandostatin is effective in lowering plasma GH and somatomedin-C and in improving clinical manifestations of acromegaly [1, 3]. In some patients, 2 daily injections were effective in lowering plasma GH significantly [1] and, in our 15 responders, 7 received 2 injec-

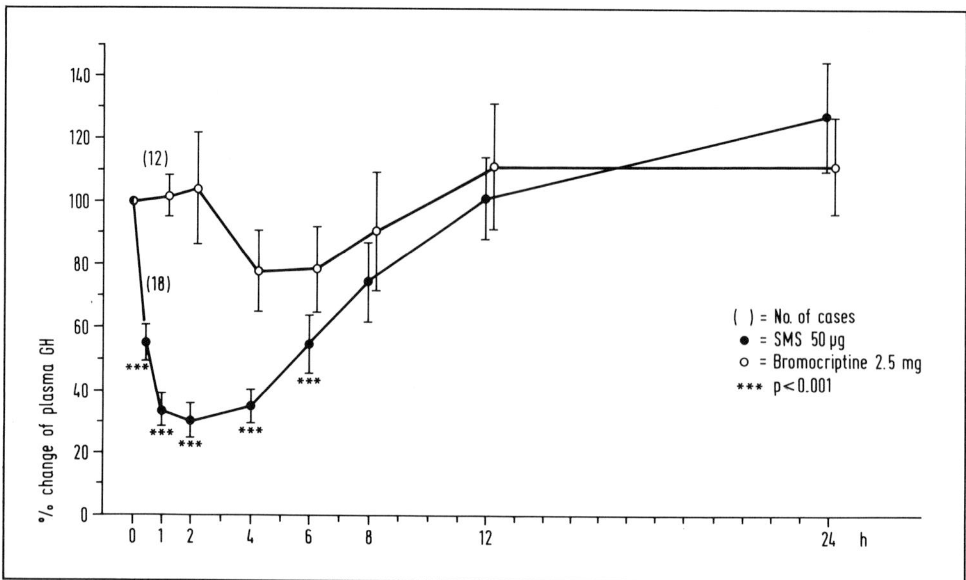

Fig. 1. Effect of a single subcutaneous injection of 50 µg Sandostatin on plasma growth hormone (GH) levels in 18 patients with acromegaly. In 12 of them, single oral administration of 2.5 mg bromocriptine was ineffective in lowering plasma GH

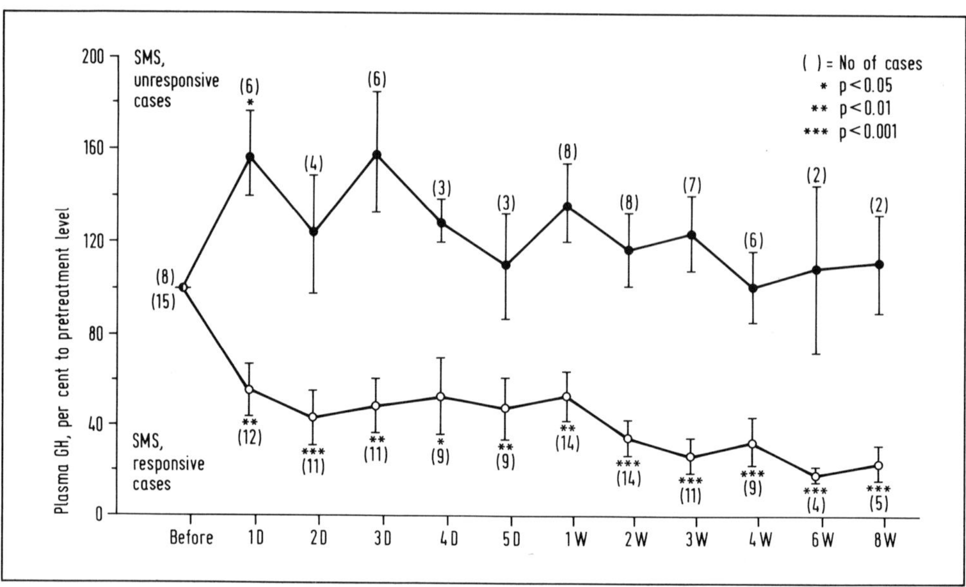

Fig. 2. Effect of 2–3 daily injections of Sandostatin on plasma growth hormone (GH) in 15 responsive cases and 8 unresponsive cases (mean values ± SEM)

tions per day. In the remaining patients, however, 3 daily injections were required to lower morning plasma GH levels signifi- cantly. Owing to the limited duration of action, however, morning GH levels below 5 ng/ml and Sm-C levels below 2 U/ml werc achicvcd in 8 and 6 patients, respectively. Incomplete suppression with 3 subcutaneous injections of 50–100 µg Sandostatin daily was also reported by Comi and Gorden [2]. An increase in dose or in frequency of injection is required in difficult cases. It is noteworthy, however, that clinical symptoms were significantly improved in most of the responsive patients without notable side effects. This suggests that repeated subcutaneous injection of Sandostatin is useful in acromegalic patients who are resistant to other therapeutic means.

References

1. Barnard LB, Gantham WG, Lamberton P, O'Dorisio TM, Jackson IMD (1986) Treatment of resistant acromegaly with a long-acting somatostatin analogue (SMS 201-995). Ann Intern Med 105:856–861
2. Comi RJ, Gorden P (1987) The response of serum growth hormone levels to the long-acting somatostatin analog SMS 201-995 in acromegaly. J Clin Endocrinol Metab 64:37–42
3. Lamberts SWJ, Uitterlinden P, Verschoor L, van Dongen KJ, Del Pozo E (1985) Long-term treatment with the somatostatin analogue SMS 201-995. N Engl J Med 313:1576–1580

19. Long-Term Treatment of Resistant Acromegaly with a Somatostatin Analog (SMS 201-995, Sandostatin®)

I. M. D. Jackson, L. Barnard, W. Cobb, M. Hein, R. Perez

Division of Endocrinology, Brown University, Rhode Island Hospital, Providence, Rhode Island, USA

The therapeutic options for acromegaly unsuitable for or unresponsive to surgery or dopaminergic agonists are limited. The short half-life ($t_{1/2}$) of natural somatostatin has precluded its use, but a new, long-acting, octapeptide analog (SMS 201-995, Sandostatin®) has shown promise [2, 4, 5]. We have reported beneficial clinical and chemical responses in 6 patients with resistant acromegaly given Sandostatin for 5−12 months [1]. This study has since been extended to include 14 patients who have received Sandostatin up to a period of 30 months.

Patients

Twelve of the 14 subjects were transsphenoidal surgical failures, and all save one had previously received external radiotherapy and/or bromocriptine. One subject with a visual field abnormality requested initial treatment with Sandostatin to see whether surgical decompression could be avoided. The clinical details of the first 6 patients studied are provided in Table 1.

Protocol

All patients gave informed consent under a research protocol approved by the Human Subjects Committee of the Rhode Island Hospital and were hospitalized for initiation of therapy with Sandostatin at 50 µg q.12 h on days 1 and 2 and 100 µg q.12 h on day 3. Through an indwelling cannula, blood was drawn at 2-hourly intervals for GH, glucose and prolactin. Following discharge from hospital, patients were seen at monthly intervals and their Sandostatin dose adjusted according to the GH and somatomedin-C levels as well as to their clinical response and freedom from side effects. High-resolution CT scans were obtained before and after Sandostatin treatment.

Results and Discussion

Following acute administration of Sandostatin, the GH level frequently showed a dramatic reduction, which was generally maintained for 6−8 h. Plasma IR-Sandostatin levels following subcutaneous injection disappeared with a $t_{1/2}$ of 119 ± 11 min for the group (Fig. 1). There was evidence that a plasma analog level − which varied in individual subjects − ranging from 70−1200 pg/ml acted as an "inhibitory threshold" on GH release. When the plasma Sandostatin fell below this concentration, GH escape occurred. On long-term therapy 7 patients have a normal somatomedin-C level on doses ranging from 50 µg q.12 h to 500 µg q.8 h. A further 5 subjects have had a significant reduction in somatomedin-C (though still raised). Of the 2 other subjects, in one there has been no change in somatomedin-C, and the other has had a persistent elevation. A reduction in tumor size of 10−33% was observed in 6 of 8 subjects in whom a repeat CT scan has thus far been performed (Fig. 2). In one patient there was a reversal of a visual field abnormality associated with a CT scan reduction in tumor size.

Symptomatic benefit has been gratifying especially in headaches and arthralgias (Table 1). Side effects (Table 1), mainly diarrhea and nausea, have not been a problem for most patients but have limited the

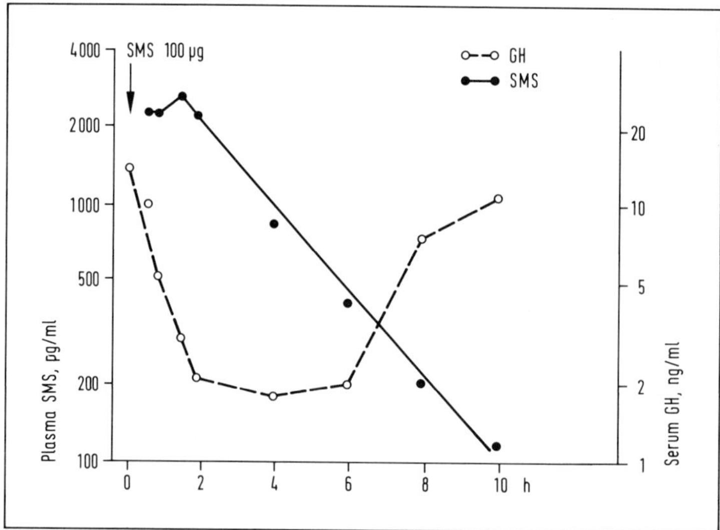

Fig. 1. Disappearance of serum growth hormone (GH) and plasma levels of Sandostatin (SMS) after subcutaneous injection of the analog in a patient with acromegaly. The half-life ($t_{1/2}$) of serum growth hormone was calculated during the first 2 h after the injection and that of Sandostatin from 2 to 10 h after administration. Note a relationship of the growth hormone levels to the plasma concentration of Sandostatin. The relatively well-maintained plasma levels of the analog during the first 2 h after administration probably reflect delayed absorption. [From 1]

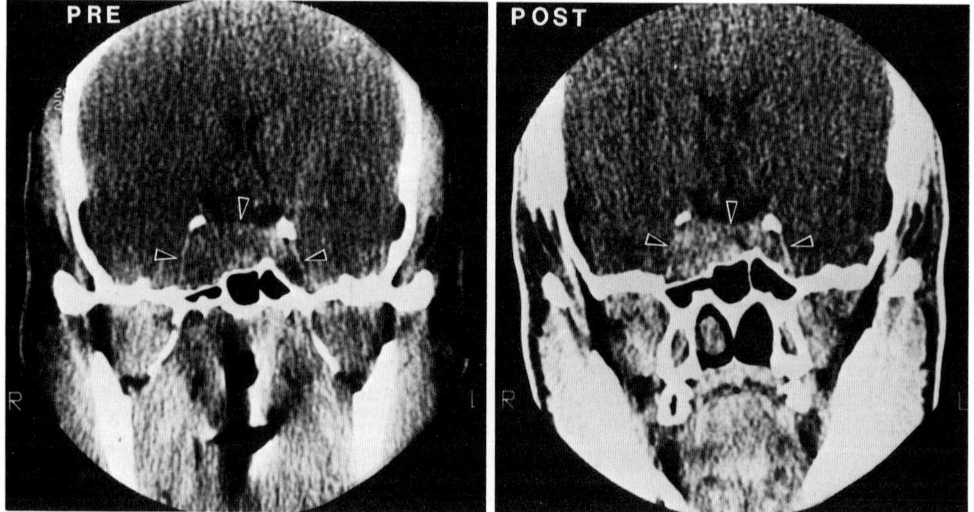

Fig. 2. CT scans pre and post 6 months' therapy with Sandostatin for acromegaly. Treatment had led to a reduction in tumor height from 1.6 to 1.4 cm

possibility of increasing the dose for some subjects. One patient, after treatment for a year, developed cholecystitis requiring surgery [3]. No major changes in carbohydrate metabolism on short- (Table 2) or long-term treatment occurred. A fall in

Table 1. Clinical response to Sandostatin. [From 1]

Patient	Age	Sex	Previous treatment	Side effects	Benefits
1	48	F	Transsphenoidal surgery × 2 and external proton beam irradiation leaving a small amount of tumor in the area of the left cavernous sinus. Bromocriptine to 60 mg q.d. with minimal benefit. On replacement with prednisone and thyroxine	Initially, several minutes of nausea post injection; transient loosening of stools over first week of starting therapy which then cleared up. No side effects now	Energy increased. "Heavy feeling" in head resolved. Shoes and rings loose. Joint pains resolved. Treatment for 1 year
2	45	M	Transsphenoidal hypophysectomy and external radiation with a residual small intrasellar tissue mass: bromocriptine up to 20 mg q.d. with limited benefit. On replacement with prednisone, thyroxine and testosterone	None	General feeling of well-being. Joint pains resolved. Treatment for 9 months
3	41	F	Transsphenoidal surgery with persistent suprasellar tumor; bromocriptine to 15 mg q.d. with no benefit. Hypogonadotropic hypogonadism	Some increase in abdominal bloating and intermittent diarrhea which was already present to some degree prior to treatment	Headache resolved. Energy increased. Joint pains decreased. Treatment for 11 months
4	24	F	Transsphenoidal hypophysectomy, transfrontal pituitary surgery, and supervoltage external radiation with residual suprasellar tumor; bromocriptine to 60 mg q.d. with no benefit. On treatment with cortisone, thyroxine and estrogen/progesterone	None	Energy increased. Fatigue lessened. Felt "happier." Lacrimation decreased. Head pain resolved. Treatment for 1 year
5	39	F	Irresectable supra-and extrasellar tumor mass. Bromocriptine up to 40 mg q.d. with some symptomatic improvement e.g. reduced headache but without change in GH or somatomedin-C levels. Pituitary function otherwise normal	None	Headache resolved. Energy increased. Treatment for 10 months
6	33	M	Transsphenoidal surgery leaving a tiny intrasellar tumor. Pituitary function otherwise normal	Transient abdominal pain following injection shortly after starting treatment. Weakness and dizziness when dose increased	Headache resolved immediately after injection. Energy and well-being improved. Treatment for 5 months

serum prolactin was observed in half the patients studied (Table 2).

In order to normalize GH levels over most of the 24-h period, Sandostatin was administered in dosages up to 1500 µg/day, fivefold that reported in other studies [2, 3, 5]. Such lower doses might account for an incomplete GH response in some of the patients described in these reports. The pharmacokinetic studies provide an explanation for patient responsiveness. Because of a $t_{1/2}$ of 2 h, in each subject the plasma SMS needs to be maintained above a certain threshold level throughout each 8-h segment after injection to normalize 24-h GH secretion. The responsiveness to Sandostatin is probably a consequence of analog binding to somatostatin receptors on the pituitary tumor [6]. We propose that the plasma concentration of the analog may reflect occupancy of somatostatin receptors and consequent inhibition of GH release.

Table 2. Effect of Sandostatin[a] on mean 24-h growth hormone, glucose, and prolactin concentration[b] over the first 3 days of treatment (mean ± SD). [From 1]

Patient	Serum growth hormone (ng/ml)		Serum prolactin (ng/ml)		Plasma glucose (mg/dl)	
	Pre-treatment	Post-treatment	Pre-treatment concentration	Post-treatment concentration	Pre-treatment concentration	Post-treatment concentration
1	48.4 ± 17.9	6.3 ± 7.3[e]	39.7 ± 3.5	25.7 ± 2.1[e]	105 ± 17	119 ± 21[c]
2	9.0 ± 2.4	1.0 ± 0.5[e]	12.6 ± 1.2	7.0 ± 1.5[e]	116 ± 20	130 ± 38
3	5.9 ± 1.9	2.3 ± 0.8[e]	27.4 ± 3.2	24.1 ± 6.3	220 ± 82	182 ± 66
4	22.5 ± 8.4	17.5 ± 7.7	5.7 ± 2.3	5.3 ± 2.5	113 ± 34	115 ± 31
5	73.9 ± 36.3	46.0 ± 26.9	26.2 ± 1.0	25.3 ± 3.8	119 ± 24	122 ± 12
6	12.0 ± 1.4	6.3 ± 4.3[e]	10.2 ± 0.8	7.3 ± 1.3[d]	108 ± 17	131 ± 46

[a] 50 or 100 µg q.12 h subcutaneously   [c] p < 0.05
[b] Samples drawn q.2 h   [d] p < 0.01
   [e] p < 0.001

Conclusions

- Sandostatin therapy is effective for long-term management of acromegaly treatment failures.
- The clinical and biochemical responses are frequently dramatic.
- The analog is relatively free from adverse clinical or biochemical side effects.

References

1. Barnard LB, Grantham WG, Lamberton MD, O'Dorisio TM, Jackson IMD (1986) Treatment of resistant acromegaly with a long-acting somatostatin analogue (SMS 201-995). Ann Intern Med 105:856–861
2. Ch'ng JLC, Sandler LM, Kraenzlin ME, Burrin JM, Joplin GF, Bloom SR (1985) Chronic treatment of acromegaly with a long-acting somatostatin analogue. Br Med J 290: 284–285
3. Jackson IMD, Barnard LB, Lamberton P (1986) Role of a long-acting somatostatin analogue (SMS 201-995) in the treatment of acromegaly. Am J Med 81 [Suppl 6B]:94–101
4. Lamberts SWJ, Oosterom R, Neufeld M, Del Pozo E (1985) The somatostatin analogue SMS 201-995 induces long-acting inhibition of growth hormone secretion without rebound hypersecretion in acromegalic patients. J Clin Endocrinol Metab 60:1161–1165
5. Lamberts SWJ, Uitterlinden P, Verschoor L, van Dongen KJ, Del Pozo E (1985) Long-term treatment of acromegaly with the somatostatin analogue SMS 201-955. N Engl J Med 313:1576–1580
6. Reubi JC, Landolt AM (1984) High density of somatostatin receptors in pituitary tumors from acromegalic patients. J Clin Endocrinol Metab 59:1148–1151

20. High-Dose, Long-Term, Continuous Subcutaneous Infusion of SMS 201-995 (Sandostatin®) in Acromegaly

S. Chatterjee, M. C. White, N. Møller, K. Hall, M. J. Dunne, E. R. Baister, P. Kendall-Taylor

Departments of Medicine and Radiology, University of Newcastle upon Tyne, UK, and Sandoz Laboratories Ltd, Basle, Switzerland

Acute and chronic studies have demonstrated the effectiveness of the long-acting somatostatin analogue SMS 201-995 (Sandostatin®) in the treatment of acromegaly. Daily doses of 100−300 µg Sandostatin given as multiple injections in most cases induce satisfactory suppression of GH release. No consistent shrinkage of the pituitary tumour has been demonstrated.

The aim of this study was to assess the long-term use of a high daily dose (1600 µg) of Sandostatin given by continuous subcutaneous infusion (CSI) with particular reference to:

(i)   reduction of serum GH and somatomedin-C levels,
(ii) shrinkage of the pituitary tumour and
(iii) patient acceptance and side effects.

We present here the data on the first seven patients to complete this ongoing study.

Patients and Methods

All the patients (4 males, 3 females, mean age 57 ± 7.7 (S.D.) years) had clinical and biochemical features of acromegaly. Five patients had previous surgery and two were considered unsuitable for surgery. Four patients had radiotherapy following their surgery. Four patients had received dopamine agonist therapy in the past, with unsatisfactory results in three of them.

Treatment and Assessment

Patients were admitted to the Investigation Unit for 4 days during which a 24-h profile of GH was obtained followed by GH response to TRH and GH response to oral glucose. A baseline CT scan of the pituitary and ultrasound of the abdomen were obtained. Treatment with Sandostatin was begun at a dose of 200 µg/day by CSI using a Graseby No. 26 pump with hourly monitoring of glucose, GH, and blood pressure for 8 h. The patients were seen weekly for reassessment and the dose was then increased by 200 µg/day increments to 1600 µg/day, which was maintained for 8 weeks. During each reassessment visit, two-hourly ambulatory GH levels were obtained from 08.00 to 16.00 h. After a total of 14 weeks of therapy, the patients were re-admitted and the pretreatment protocol was repeated.

Results

Five of the 7 patients responded well to Sandostatin and the data are shown. One patient who also responded was withdrawn because of adverse effects. One patient did not respond to the treatment as judged by absence of change in mean 24-h GH levels, and GH response to oral glucose or TRH (data not shown).

The 24-h GH profile was significantly lower at all time points after treatment (Fig. 1). The individual GH peaks were attenuated after treatment in all five patients. There was a marked lowering of GH after 1 week of treatment with 400 µg/day of Sandostatin (Fig. 2); somatomedin-C was simultaneously reduced into the low normal range (normal range 12−48 nmol/l). As the study was designed to assess the effects of high-dose therapy the dose was increased at weekly intervals, but no further drop in GH or Sm-C levels was noted. The GH response to oral glucose was markedly reduced (Table 1). The plasma glucose at 90 min was

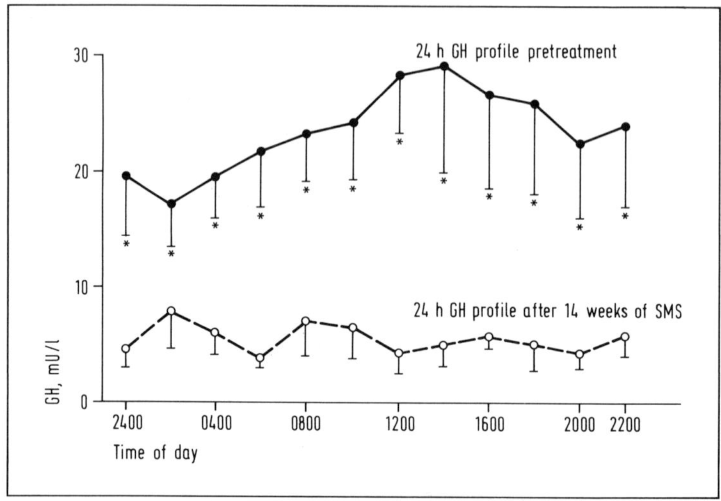

Fig. 1. Difference in mean 24-h growth hormone (GH) levels before and after treatment. All the post-treatment values are lower than (p ≤ 0.04) pretreatment values

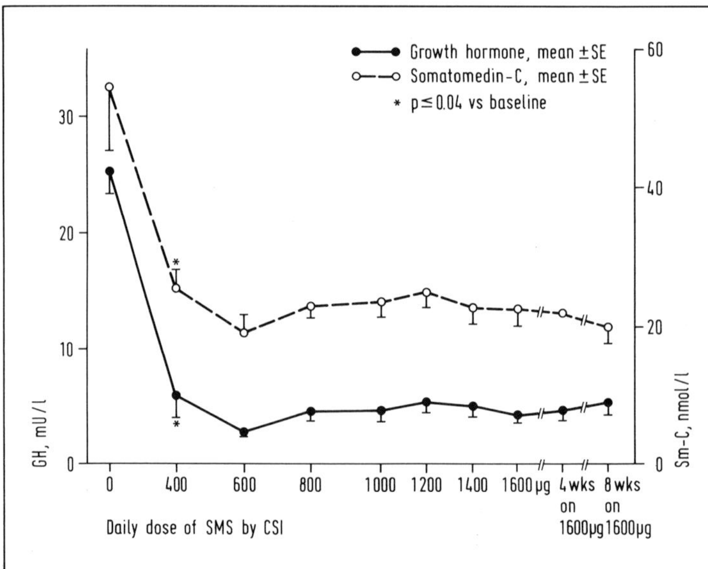

Fig. 2. Fall of mean ambulatory growth hormone (GH) (2-hourly samples from 08.00 to 16.00 h) and somatomedin-C levels. All the values are different (p ≤ 0.04) from baseline. n = 6 at baseline and 400 µg, n = 5 at other points

Table 1. OGTT: GH, insulin and glucose responses to 75 g oral glucose before and after 14 weeks of Sandostatin treatment. Data from 5 patients who completed the study and responded to treatment

Min	GH (mU/l)		Insulin (mU/l)		Glucose (nmol/l)	
	pre	post	pre	post	pre	post
0	20.6 ± 9.0	$4.0 \pm 0.9^*$	3.8 ± 0.4	2.0 ± 0.7	4.8 ± 0.5	4.5 ± 0.2
30	24.8 ± 10.3	3.5 ± 0.8	19.6 ± 2.1	$8.5 \pm 2.0^*$	7.6 ± 1.1	8.0 ± 2.1
60	23.8 ± 7.3	$3.8 \pm 1.8^*$	24.4 ± 9.7	16.3 ± 3.2	10.2 ± 1.8	10.2 ± 1.0
90	27.9 ± 6.4	$3.6 \pm 1.3^*$	23.8 ± 5.2	22.3 ± 6.7	8.2 ± 1.6	$10.5 \pm 1.2^*$
120	29.7 ± 6.3	$3.8 \pm 1.4^*$	24.5 ± 3.6	17.7 ± 6.0	6.1 ± 1.5	7.2 ± 3.8

* p < 0.05

Table 2. GH response to TRH 200 µg i.v. (data from 5 patients)

Min	Pre-SMS GH mU/l	After 14 weeks GH mU/l	
0	27.8 ± 6.2	12.7 ± 6.3	p = .01
20	95.1 ± 31.1	12.2 ± 4.0	p = .04
60	39.4 ± 8.6	7.9 ± 3.0	p = .02

higher after treatment (p = 0.03), while the plasma insulin was lower at 30 min (p = 0.04). A trend towards lower insulin and higher glucose values was noted throughout the post-treatment OGTT. There was no clinical evidence of worsened glucose tolerance or rise in HbA$_1$C while on treatment (Table 2).

There was no CT scan evidence of diminished tumour size in any patient.

Adverse Effects

One patient with hypopituitarism was withdrawn from the study after 12 days because of vomiting and abdominal cramps leading to hypoadrenalism. Five patients, including the non-responder, reported mild flatulence and soft stools 1−2 times a day, which improved during the course of treatment. One patient had no side effects. There was no abnormality of thyroid function. The withdrawn patient, who was the only diabetic responder, was able to stop taking sulphonylurea and biguanide tablets while remaining euglycaemic on Sandostatin. In all patients liver and gallbladder ultrasound remained normal after 14 weeks. Routine biochemistry remained normal throughout.

The patients had no problems in handling their infusion pumps. All the 5 responders felt better while on it. At the end of 14 weeks, 4 of these patients chose to continue treatment with Sandostatin. There was no local skin reaction, except in one patient who inadvertently used the same infusion site for 7 days.

Discussion

Using a CSI mode of delivery, doses of up to 1600 µg/d could be safely used if required. Sandostatin was well tolerated in 6 out of 7 patients and was effective in lowering GH levels in 6 out of the 7 patients. The lowering of GH and Sm-C levels was evident within 1 week in the responders, and the non-responder could be identified within 1 week. GH peaks were abolished and Sm-C reduced to low normal levels. The GH response to glucose was not normalized after treatment according to our previously established criteria. There were small, clinically unimportant, changes in glucose and insulin levels to a glucose challenge.

Though there was no change in tumour size, small differences would be hard to discern in this group of patients, most of whom have had previous surgery/radiotherapy.

This study was not designed to determine the minimum effective dose of Sandostatin though our data would suggest that doses greater than 400 or 600 µg/d do not confer added benefit or add to the toxicity. If gastrointestinal side effects are severe, there is a definite possibility of increased glucocorticoid requirements in patients on replacement therapy.

21. Long-Term Therapy of Acromegaly with SMS 201-995 (Sandostatin®)

D. Killinger, J. Gonzalez

Department of Medicine, University of Toronto, Toronto, Ontario, Canada

SMS 201-995 (Sandostatin®), a long-acting analogue of somatostatin, has been shown to be effective in lowering growth hormone (GH) levels in patients with acromegaly [1, 2]. Suppression of GH levels persists for 6 to 8 h and a treatment schedule of two or three daily injections is required to maintain optimum suppression. In the present study, 2 patients who had been unsuccessfully treated by surgery or surgery and pituitary irradiation were treated with Sandostatin for 12 to 18 months and clinical and laboratory parameters were followed to determine the efficacy of treatment.

Patients

Patient 1 is a 50-year-old male who was initially treated for severe acromegaly in 1972 with proton beam irradiation. In 1981 he was investigated and found to have a stage III adenoma with basal GH levels of 110 to 150 µg/l and normal prolactin levels. Transsphenoidal surgery decreased GH levels to 40 to 60 µg/l and treatment with bromocriptine up to 20 mg daily resulted in no further decrease in GH levels. There was no change in subjective complaints or clinical findings of gross acromegaly, and headaches and arthritis became progressively more debilitating. Treatment with Sandostatin began in May 1986.

Patient 2 is a 40-year-old female who was initially investigated in 1978 and found to have elevated GH (60 µg/l) and prolactin (58 µg/l) levels. Transsphenoidal surgery decreased GH levels to 20 to 30 µg/l and prolactin levels to 20 µg/l. Pituitary pathology revealed a mixed GH and prolactin cell adenoma. Treatment with bromocriptine lowered prolactin levels and the patient became pregnant. A normal female infant was born in 1981. In 1986 the patient returned and GH levels were found to be 40 to 60 µg/l with prolactin levels of 12 µg/l. She was complaining of severe headaches, progressive thyroid enlargement and progressive facial changes.

Results

Figure 1 shows the response of GH levels in patient 1 to different doses of Sandostatin. A 50 µg dose injected subcutaneously resulted in an 80% fall in GH levels with maximum effect by 2 h. Doses of 200 and 300 µg of Sandostatin did not result in a further decrease in GH levels, but suppression was somewhat more sustained.

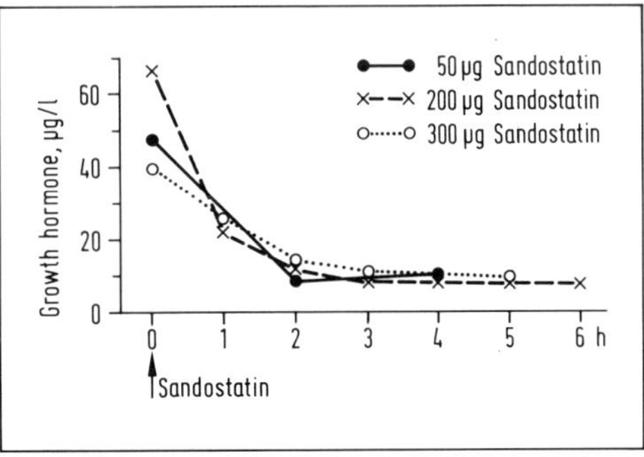

Fig. 1. Effect of dose of Sandostatin on growth hormone levels

Figure 2 shows GH levels taken hourly over 48 h with Sandostatin administered at a dose of 200 µg every 8 h for the first 24 h and 250 µg every 8 h for the second 24 h. The difference in dosage did not produce a signifi-

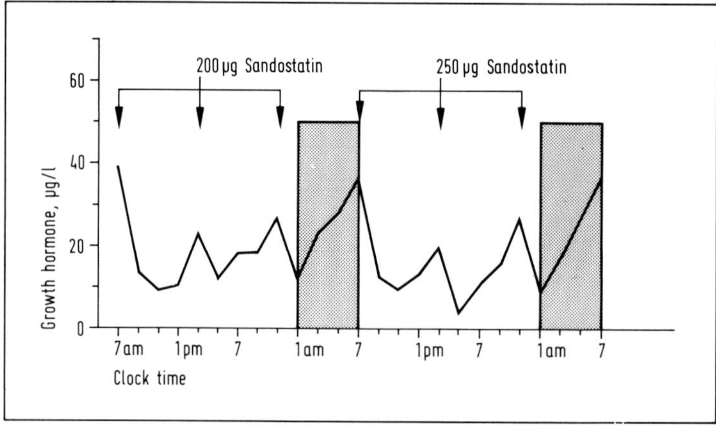

Fig. 2. Growth hormone levels on 200 µg and 250 µg of Sandostatin every 8 h

cant difference in GH suppression. There was a partial escape prior to each injection and the nocturnal rise appeared to be somewhat greater than at other times of the day.

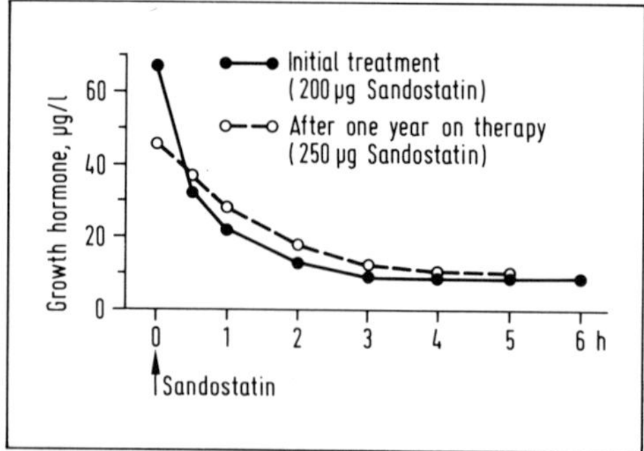

Fig. 3. Growth hormone response to Sandostatin prior to, and after, 1 year of treatment

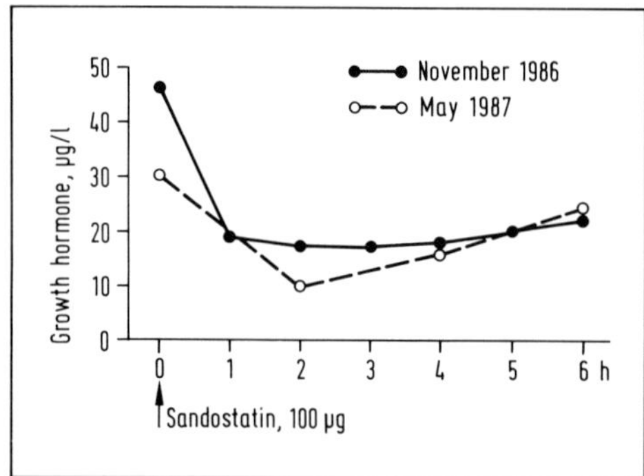

Fig. 4. The effect of Sandostatin before and after 6 months of treatment

GH levels did not suppress to normal at any time throughout the study.

Figure 3 shows a comparison of GH suppression in patient 1 at the start of the study and after treatment for 1 year with Sandostatin 250 µg three times per day. Figure 4 shows a similar study before and after 6 months of treatment with 100 µg Sandostatin three times per day in patient 2. In both subjects, there was no decrease in GH suppressibility during the treatment period.

In both patients, there was dramatic relief of the headache with the first injection. Patient 1 noted return of his headache prior to each injection and there was a good correlation with the rise in GH levels. Both patients developed transient diarrhea and abdominal cramps which cleared while still on the medication. No other side effects were noted.

Discussion

In both of the patients, previously treated unsuccessfully by surgery or surgery plus irradiation, Sandostatin decreased GH levels dramatically, although in neither patient were GH levels decreased to normal. Increasing the dose of Sandostatin from 50 to 300 µg per injection did not result in a progressive decrease in GH levels. The effectiveness of Sandostatin was sustained during the treatment periods of 6 to 12 months and there was no adverse effect on fasting blood sugars. As reported by Sandler et al. [4] and Richmond et al. [3], the relief of headache was dramatic and occurred shortly after the onset of therapy. The gastrointestinal side effects, which occurred in both patients, subsided without treatment.

In these patients, Sandostatin was an effective, well-tolerated therapy which reduced GH levels by 75 to 80% and resulted in dramatic relief of headaches and a progressive improvement in soft tissue changes of acromegaly.

Acknowledgments: The authors would like to thank Patricia Leahy and the staff of the Clinical Investigation Unit of the Wellesley Hospital for carrying out these studies and assisting in the follow up of these patients. The study was supported by a grant from the Whitney Foundation

References

1. Ch'ng JLC, Sandler LM, Kraenzlin ME, Burrin JM, Joplin GF, Bloom SR (1985) Chronic treatment of acromegaly with a long-acting somatostatin analogue. Br Med J 290: 284−285
2. Lamberts SWJ, Oosterman R, Neufeld M, Del Pozo E (1985) The somatostatin analogue SMS 201-995 induced long-acting inhibition of growth hormone secretion without rebound hypersecretion in acromegalic patients. J Clin Endocrinol Metab 60:1161−1165
3. Richmond W, Seviour PW, Teal TK, Elkeles RS (1987) Analgesic effect of somatostatin analogue (octreotide) in headache associated with pituitary tumours. Br Med J 295:247−248
4. Sandler LM, Burrin JM, Williams G, Joplin GF, Carr DH, Bloom SR (1987) Effective long-term treatment of acromegaly with a long-acting somatostatin analogue (SMS 201-995). Clin Endocrinol 26:85−95

22. Successful Treatment of Ophthalmoplegia in Acromegaly with the Somatostatin Analogue SMS 201-995 (Sandostatin®)

P. A. van Liessum, G. F. F. M. Pieters, A. R. M. M. Hermus, A. G. H. Smals,
P. W. C. Kloppenborg

Department of Medicine, Division of Endocrinology, University Hospital, University of Nijmegen,
The Netherlands
Correspondence:
P. A. van Liessum, Department of Medicine, Division of Endocrinology, University Hospital, P.O.
Box 9101, 6500 HB Nijmegen, The Netherlands

Ophthalmoplegia without visual field defects is a rare complication of pituitary adenomas nowadays. The first treatment is often neurosurgical decompression, though results are conflicting. We report on an acromegalic patient whose ophthalmoplegia completely resolved during treatment with the long-acting somatostatin analogue SMS 201-995 (Sandostatin®), which has been shown to have a long-acting inhibitory effect on plasma GH in patients with acromegaly without rebound hypersecretion [3–5].

Case Report

In a 60-year-old woman, twenty months before admission, acromegaly without sellar enlargement or visual field defects was diagnosed. This was confirmed by elevated basal growth hormone (GH) levels (11–18 mU/l, RIA) which did not decline during an oral glucose tolerance test. She was then treated with bromocriptine 2.5 mg three times daily. Two months before admission diabetes mellitus was detected, which was treated with diet and glibenclamide medication. During this period GH levels on bromocriptine therapy were at a mean level of 20 mU/l. This was considered as continuing activity of acromegaly. Sandostatin therapy or neurosurgery were proposed, but she postponed the decision.

Four weeks prior to admission she noticed a predominantly right-sided constant hyperesthesia of the hairy scalp and frontal headache developed. Four days before she was admitted, pain around the right eye also occurred, followed next day by diplopia, dizziness and nausea. On admission there were also complaints of paresthesias predominantly on the right side of the face and the back of the tongue and palate, as well as toothache in the right upper jaw, although she was edentulous.

Physical examination showed no acute distress. There was a nearly total ptosis of the right eye and complete palsy of the right oculomotor nerve and an incomplete palsy of the right abducens. Visual fields were normal. Laboratory investigation revealed a glucose level of 10.7 mmol/l. Further routine blood tests were unremarkable.

A high-resolution CT scan of the brain showed an intrasellar tumour predominantly localized in the right part of the sella with some bulging to the suprasellar region and slight parasellar extension to the right. There was an even distribution of contrast in the pituitary without impressive asymmetrical filling of the cavernous sinuses (Fig. 1A).

Therapy was started the day after admission with Sandostatin three times 100 μg s.c. per day. On day 3 the pain around the eye disappeared, followed by complete resolution of complaints and symptoms within less than three weeks. GH levels during treatment decreased to a mean value of 4 mU/l, measured 4 h after Sandostatin injection.

A second CT scan, performed three weeks after starting therapy, showed shrinkage of the tumour established by decline of bulging towards the suprasellar region. Only a slight parasellar reduction was seen on the right side (Fig. 1B).

Until now (follow up: seven months) she is continuing Sandostatin treatment and remains well without symptoms.

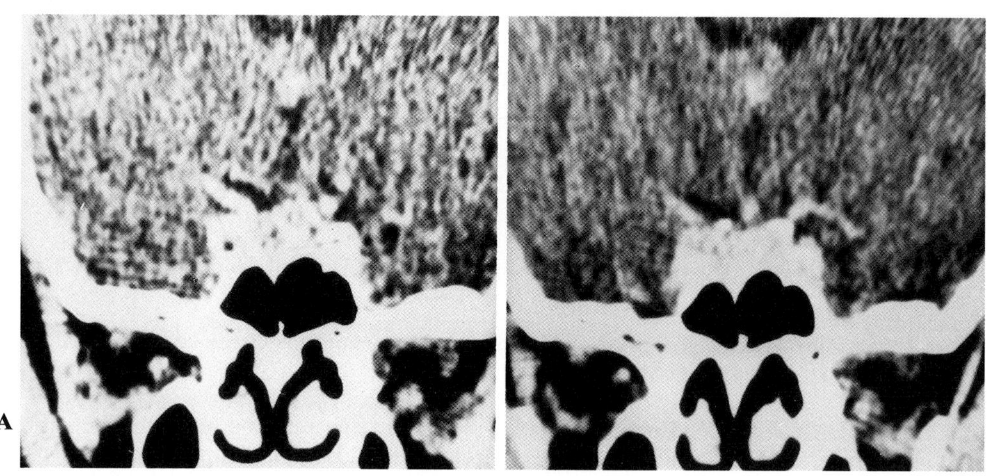

Fig. 1. High-resolution CT scan of the pituitary region before **(A)** and after **(B)** three weeks of treatment with Sandostatin. See text for further comment

Discussion

We strongly believe that this patient suffered from eye symptoms due to tumour growth, which also explains her rather slowly developing complaints, the development of overt diabetes and the rise of GH levels despite bromocriptine therapy. This lack of an acute event together with an even distribution of contrast in the pituitary excludes pituitary apoplexy as an explanation.

In comparison with the frequent shrinkage of prolactinomas treated with bromocriptine, only rarely is this described during such treatment of acromegaly [6]. However, during Sandostatin therapy tumour diminution has been reported in 60% of 27 acromegalics [2], while one had also relief of ophthalmoplegia [3]. This latter patient had a recurrence after stopping self-administration of the drug and improved again after restarting treatment. In our patient, only a slight parasellar reduction of the tumour on the right side was demonstrated by CT scan three weeks after starting Sandostatin, but visual improvement has previously been shown to precede shrinkage of pituitary adenomas [1]. Larger series are awaited to see whether tumour diminution occurs regularly during Sandostatin therapy and whether it will be the therapy of choice in acromegaly with mechanical complications

of the pituitary adenoma.

In conclusion, this report suggests an important therapeutic role for Sandostatin in ophthalmoplegia due to pituitary GH-producing adenomas.

Acknowledgements: The authors thank H. O. M. Thijssen and J. L. Merkx (Dept of Neuroradiology) for their comment on the CT scans and Mrs. W. Straten for excellent secretarial assistance.

References

1. Chiodini P, Liuzzi A, Cozzi R, Verde G, Oppizzi G, Dallabonzana D, Spelta B, Silvestrini F, Borghi G, Luccarelli G, Rainer E, Horowski R (1981) Size reduction of macroprolactinomas by bromocriptine or lisuride treatment. J Clin Endocrinol Metab 53: 737−743
2. Jackson IMD, Barnard LB, Lamberton P (1986) Role of a long-acting somatostatin analogue (SMS 201-995) in the treatment of acromegaly. Am J Med 81 [Suppl 6B]:94−101
3. Lamberts SWJ, Uitterlinden P, Verschoor L, van Dongen KJ, Del Pozo E (1985) Long-term treatment of acromegaly with the somatostatin analogue SMS 201-995. N Engl J Med 313: 1576−1580
4. Pieters GFFM, Smals AGH, Kloppenborg PWC (1986) Long-term treatment of acromegaly with the somatostatin analogue SMS 201-995. N Engl J Med 314:1391
5. Plewe G, Beyer J, Krause U, Neufeld M, Del Pozo E (1984) Long-acting and selective sup-

pression of growth hormone secretion by somatostatin analogue SMS 201-995 in acromegaly. Lancet II:782−784

6. Wass JAH, Moult PJA, Thorner MO, Dacie JE, Charlesworth M, Jones AE, Besser GM (1979) Reduction of pituitary-tumour size in patients with prolactinomas and acromegaly treated with bromocriptine with or without radiotherapy. Lancet II:66−69

23. Sandostatin® (SMS 201-995) in the Treatment of Acromegaly

M. L. Vance, D. L. Kaiser, M. O. Thorner

Division of Endocrinology, Department of Internal Medicine, University of Virginia School of Medicine, Charlottesville, Virginia, USA

Acromegaly, a disorder of excessive growth hormone (GH) secretion, is most commonly caused by a pituitary adenoma and is usually treated by surgical resection. However, as with other types of pituitary tumors, the cure rate usually reflects the size of the tumor, i.e., complete resection of a macroadenoma (>10 mm diameter) and cure occurs in only a minority. Additionally, a rare cause of acromegaly, pituitary stimulation by an ectopic tumor which secretes growth hormone releasing hormone (GHRH), may not be cured by surgical resection if metastases are present. Frequently patients with active disease following primary surgical therapy require additional treatment, either pituitary radiation or medical therapy. Since radiotherapy may not be effective for several years after the treatment, there is a need for other therapeutic modalities. Dopamine agonists, bromocriptine; lisuride, pergolide, have been used to treat acromegalics and are associated with symptomatic improvement despite incomplete suppression of GH secretion. Thus the development of another approach to a medical treatment of acromegaly is needed. Growth hormone secretion is primarily regulated by two hypothalamic peptides, GHRH which stimulates, and somatostatin which inhibits, release. The development of a long-acting somatostatin analog which acts more selectively on the somatotrope than on the pancreas is a theoretically ideal compound for medical therapy of acromegaly. Sandostatin® is an octapeptide somatostatin analog which may fulfill these criteria and is currently undergoing clinical trials in Europe and North America. We have treated 8 acromegalic patients with Sandostatin for up to 36 months and report the results here.

Methods

Eight acromegalic patients were enrolled in the study which was approved by the Human Investigation Committee. Criteria for inclusion were an elevated serum somatomedin-C (normal $0.34 - 2.2$ U/ml) and lack of GH suppression to <2 ng/ml after ingestion of 100 g of glucose. Three patients received no prior therapy for acromegaly (patients 2, 3, 4), one of whom has ectopic GHRH secretion from metastatic carcinoid (patient 2). Patients 5–8 had undergone transsphenoidal surgery and patient 1 had undergone surgery and radiotherapy. Two patients (3 and 6) had impaired vision and visual field defects. On the control day and subsequent treatment evaluation days, serum GH levels were measured either every 20 min for 12 h or every hour for 24 h. Blood glucose was measured every hour. Patients were evaluated every 3 months during treatment. The initial SMS 201-995 dose was either 100 µg every 12 h or 100 µg every 8 h. Doses were increased to a maximum of 500 µg every 8 h if incomplete GH suppression occurred with a smaller dose. The duration of therapy was from 1 to 36 months. The patient with ectopic GHRH secretion (patient 2) was placed on a continuous subcutaneous infusion of Sandostatin, 1000 µg/day, after 2 years of intermittent therapy.

Results

All reported an improvement in overall sense of well-being and diminished sweating. All developed acholic stools during the first 1–2 weeks of therapy; stool color then returned to normal. Some patients reported

Table 1. Mean serum GH (ng/ml) and somatomedin-C (U/ml) levels before and during Sandostatin therapy in 8 acromegalics. The dose of Sandostatin is shown in the last column

Patient	Pre	On Rx (Month)	Pre	On Rx	Dose (µg)
		GH		**Sm-C**	
1	15.6	1.6 (36)	7.3	1.5	500 t.i.d.
2*	31.5	9.8 (36)	5.9	1.0	1000/24 h
3*	14.3	6.8 (24)	3.4	3.2	500 t.i.d.
4*	81.9	11.2 (21)	7.0	2.2	500 t.i.d.
5	5.8	1.5 (18)	2.6	0.6	500 t.i.d.
6	9.2	0.6 (15)	6.3	0.3	500 t.i.d.
7	27.5	9.6 (6)	18.3	2.5	500 t.i.d.
8	15.8	8.4 (1)	4.3	1.6	100 t.i.d.

* Sandostatin as primary therapy

stinging at the injection site which decreased when the injection was given slowly. Otherwise, there were no adverse effects. The 2 patients with visual field defects had improvement in vision and reduction in tumor size as shown by CT scan. Patient 3 had improvement in vision within 6 days of beginning therapy; visual acuity was 20/400 OD, 20/50 OS before treatment and was 20/50 OD and 20/25 OS on day 6. Patient 6 had a pretreatment visual acuity of 20/60 OD and no light perception OS. After 6 months of therapy the visual acuity was 20/30 OD and + hand motion OS.

Serum GH levels declined in all patients during Sandostatin therapy. Table 1 shows the mean serum GH and serum somatomedin-C levels before treatment and at the most recent evaluation. Mean serum GH levels decreased by 69% for the group. The duration of GH suppression after a Sandostatin dose was, on average, 5 to 6 h. While GH levels increased prior to the next dose, most patients did not have a marked "rebound" increase. The patient with ectopic GHRH secretion had a decrease in both GH and GHRH levels during treatment. This suppression was more pronounced during continuous subcutaneous than during intermittent therapy. However, complete suppression of GH and GHRH levels did not occur. Serum somatomedin-C levels also declined during therapy; a 70% reduction occurred for the group. Postprandial hyperglycemia (usually in the morning) occurred in 6 patients; three of these are diabetic.

Conclusion

Sandostatin is effective therapy for both pituitary-dependent and ectopic GHRH-mediated acromegaly. The somatostatin analog is well tolerated and, in this group of patients, is not associated with significant side effects. From this small number of patients, it is not possible to determine whether the progressive decrease in GH levels is a result of duration of therapy or of increasing dosage.

24. Somatostatin Octapeptide (SMS 201-995, Sandostatin®) in the Medical Treatment of Acromegaly

J. A. H. Wass[1], K. Davidson[2], S. Medbak[2], G. M. Besser[1]

Departments of Endocrinology[1] and Chemical Endocrinology[2], St Bartholomew's Hospital, London, UK

In current studies we have aimed to establish 1) that Sandostatin® has a prolonged intravenous half-life in man; 2) that it causes suppression of growth hormone levels in acromegaly; 3) the dose necessary to achieve this suppression; 4) whether Sandostatin works in patients unresponsive to bromocriptine and whether there is any additive effect of using both drugs simultaneously; 5) whether there is nocturnal escape of growth hormone secretion on Sandostatin in comparison with bromocriptine and 6) the effects and side effects of long-term treatment, including an assessment of pituitary tumour size.

1) We have established a specific radioimmunoassay for Sandostatin which does not cross-react with native somatostatin. Studies of the half-life in 3 normal subjects showed that this was prolonged to a mean of 110 min.

2) A comparison of the intravenous administration of 0.2 µg/min of Sandostatin was made with somatostatin (2 µg/min) and saline in 3 patients. Prolonged suppression of growth hormone was achieved with Sandostatin compared with native somatostatin where growth hormone levels began to rise after a few minutes. In contrast, the suppression of insulin during Sandostatin and somatostatin infusion was similar and not greatly prolonged by Sandostatin.

3) Single-dose comparisons in untreated acromegalics given saline, 50, 100, 200 and 400 µg subcutaneously showed increasing suppression of growth hormone levels. After 50 µg, growth hormone levels began to rise at 3 h. After 200 µg they did not rise for 9 h.

4) A study of 8 acromegalic patients on no treatment, bromocriptine 10−40 mg/day and Sandostatin 150−600 µg daily was carried out and showed that in all but one patient control of growth hormone levels was better with Sandostatin. Addition of bromocriptine had no further effect on GH levels.

5) In a comparison of daytime and nighttime growth hormone values in 12 patients before and on Sandostatin (150−600 µg/day) (6) or bromocriptine (10−40 mg daily) (6) growth hormone values were well suppressed throughout the whole 24-h period in 4 patients on Sandostatin. Two patients showed escape during the night. In the bromocriptine-treated patients no escape was seen during night-time.

6) During long-term treatment in 14 patients given 200−600 µg daily (2−3 doses) for 11−29 months, growth hormone levels fell in all patients studied. Mean levels before treatment ranged from 13−90 mU/l. On treatment, growth hormone levels ranged from 2−35 mU/l and they were below 20 mU/l in all but one patient. No deterioration in carbohydrate tolerance occurred. Prolactin levels fell from above normal to normal in one patient. In the other patients no change in prolactin secretion was seen. Side effects were noted in some patients. Nine noticed mild abdominal pain, 6 mild diarrhea. Over this period there was no change in the hematology, urea and electrolytes, liver function tests, serum iron and folate, Vitamin D, prothrombin time or HBA_1C. In 5 out of 14 there was a decrease in the size of the pituitary tumour, and in one this was marked. Sweating decreased in 12 out of 12 patients, headaches improved in 11 out of 12, hand size decreased in 13 out of 14 and hypertension (<90 mm mercury diastolic) became normal in 3 out of 6.

Conclusions

When compared with natural somatostatin, Sandostatin has a prolonged circulating half-life in man. Sandostatin causes prolonged growth hormone suppression in acromegaly. Subcutaneous administration of 50 µg causes less prolonged suppression of growth hormone than does 200 µg. The drug is effective in patients resistant to treatment with bromocriptine. Nocturnal escape of growth hormone secretion can occur, but this may be a problem of inadequate dosage. Growth hormone levels fall in the majority of patients treated. Symptoms improve in the majority of patients, and no serious adverse effects have been seen so far. Tumour size can decrease, but this is not clinically significant in the patients we have studied.

25a. SMS 201-995 (Sandostatin®) Treatment of Therapy-Resistant Acromegaly

J. Schopohl, O. A. Müller, K. von Werder

Medizinische Klinik Innenstadt, Universität München, FRG

Since long-acting somatostatin preparations have become available, they have been used for the treatment of acromegaly with great success [1, 2, 5, 6]. The greatest experience has been obtained with the octapeptide analogue, Sandostatin®, which leads at a dosage of 50 µg s.c. to a significant decrease of GH levels lasting up to 8 h [3, 6]. Dosages of 3 × 50 or 3 × 100 µg Sandostatin s.c. were shown to normalize GH secretion in 90% of acromegalic patients [2, 3] without serious side effects on carbohydrate metabolism and the gastrointestinal tract [1, 3–5, 7].

We have treated 7 selected patients with Sandostatin (Table 1); of these 2 had ectopic GHRH production with acromegaly and gigantism, respectively. Both patients had metastatic GHRH-producing tumours and in both patients Sandostatin not only suppressed GH but also GHRH levels. One patient has been treated now for more than 3 years resulting in a significant shrinkage of liver metastases, although the Sandostatin dosage had to be increased up to 700 µg/day to ensure complete suppression of GH and GHRH levels (Fig. 1).

The 5 other patients had large invasive somatotropic tumours, one of them being inoperable because of a suprasellar extending tumour leading to blockade of foramen Monroe (Table 1). The other 4 patients had been operated by transsphenoidal or transfrontal approach 2 or 3 times, respectively, and had received postoperative radiotherapy and dopamine agonists without success. In all 5 patients Sandostatin treatment led to further decrease of GH levels, although normalization of GH levels was only achieved in the 3 patients who had basal GH

Table 1. Sandostatin treatment in resistant acromegaly

Patient	Pathology	Previous therapy	Sandostatin (µg/day)	Duration (month)	GH (ng/ml) before	on SMS
A. S.	Macroadenoma	1 × transsphenoidal-op, 1 × transfrontal-op	1000	8	60	5
M. S.	Macroadenoma	3 × transsphenoidal-op, rad., DA-agon.	750*	18	160	30
H. A.	Macroadenoma	3 × transsphenoidal-op, rad., DA-agon.	200	24	25	2.5
K. R.	Macroadenoma	2 × transsphenoidal-op, rad., DA-agon.	300	10	45	5
M. M.	Giant adenoma with hydrocephalus int.	inoperable	600−1200*	3	350	50
B. S.	Metastasizing GHRH-oma	transsphenoidal-op, laparotomy	700*	40	25	<1
B. M.	Metastasizing GHRH-oma	thoracotomy	100	0.5	10	<1

* CSI

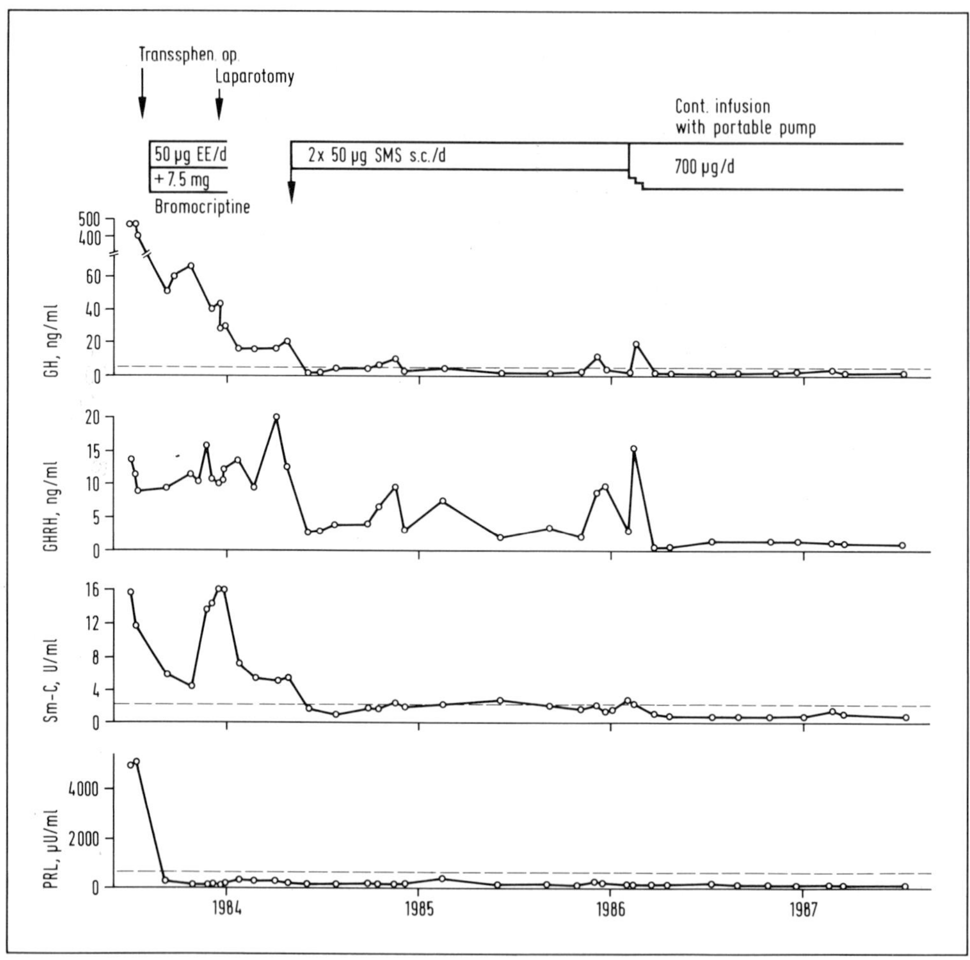

Fig. 1. Growth hormone (GH), growth hormone releasing hormone (GHRH), somatomedin-C and prolactin (PRL) levels before and after transsphenoidal surgery, laparotomy and during chronic Sandostatin treatment in a 14-year-old female patient with a GHRH-producing foregut carcinoid. GH levels fell from above 400 to 50 ng/ml after transsphenoidal-op and showed a further decrease after laparotomy though GHRH levels were not influenced. After starting Sandostatin treatment GH levels were suppressed and GHRH levels fell by 75%. Somatomedin-C levels which were already suppressed during a short period of estrogen treatment were normalized during treatment with Sandostatin. However, the dosage had to be increased up to 700 µg/day to achieve and maintain complete GH and GHRH suppression. This dosage was tolerated without side effects when given by continuous subcutaneous infusion (CSI)

levels less than 100 ng/ml before Sandostatin therapy (Table 1). Three patients received daily dosages of Sandostatin exceeding 500 µg/day, one patient up to 1500 µg/day which could only be administered without side effects by using a portable pump for continuous subcutaneous infusion (CSI) of Sandostatin. Patients who had not tolerated a bolus injection of 100 µg Sando-

statin showed no side effects when dosages from 700 up to 1500 µg Sandostatin were given by CSI. In one of the patients receiving Sandostatin (Fig. 2), higher GH levels were observed when the same dose (1500 µg Sandostatin) was given subcutaneously in comparison with i.v. administration. This suggests incomplete absorption of Sandostatin when the latter is given in larger vol-

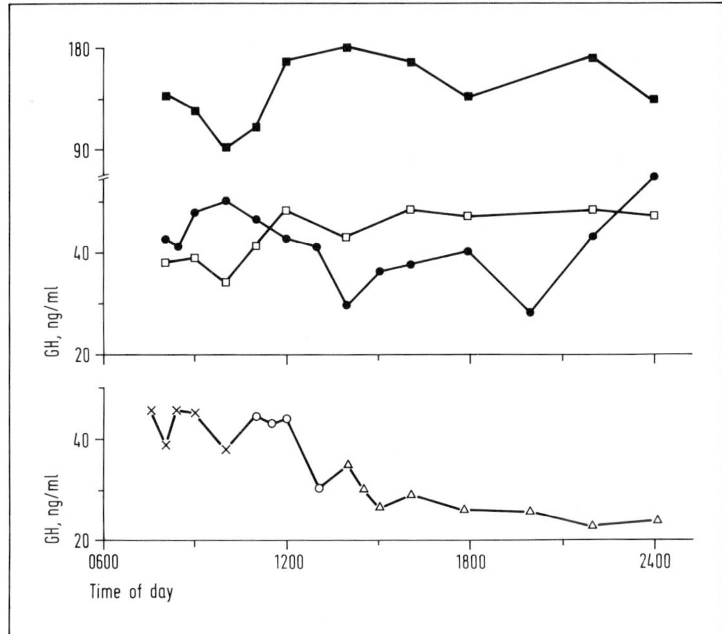

Fig. 2. Twenty-four-hour growth hormone (GH) profiles from a 26-year-old patient after 3 transsphenoidal operations, radiation and under 30 mg bromocriptine/day, on 750 µg Sandostatin/24 h given by CSI, 1500 µg by CSI and on increasing Sandostatin dosages administered intravenously. All dosages were tolerated without side effects. A clear-cut fall of GH levels was observed with 750 µg Sandostatin/24 h although no normalization was seen. Whereas there was only a slight further decrease after doubling subcutaneous dosage, a constant further fall of GH levels between 20 and 25 ng/ml could be observed with i.v. infusion of 1500 µg Sandostatin/24 h. This suggests that dosages above 750 µg/day are probably not entirely resorbed due to the large volume (between 1.5 and 3 ml/24 h). ■ = control; ● = 750 µg/24 h s.c.; □ = 1500 µg/24 h s.c. Intravenous administration rate: × = 375 µg/24 h; ○ = 750 µg/24 h; △ = 1500 µg/24 h

umes (3 ml) subcutaneously.

None of the 7 patients (therapy duration up to 40 months) developed gallstones or showed deterioration of carbohydrate tolerance or gastrointestinal side effects.

Our results show a good effect of Sandostatin in lowering GH levels also in those patients who after previous conventional therapy were not cured and in patients with the rare GHRH-producing tumours which could not be removed surgically.

References

1. Chiodini PG, Cozzi R, Dallabonzana D, Oppizzi G, Verde G, Petroncini M, Liuzzi A, Del Pozo E (1987) Medical treatment of acromegaly with SMS 201-995, a Somatostatin analog: A comparison with bromocriptine. J Clin Endocrinol Metab 64:447

2. Comi RJ, Gorden P (1987) The response of serum growth hormone levels to long-acting somatostatin analog SMS 201-995 in acromegaly. J Clin Endocrinol Metab 64:37

3. Lamberts SWJ, Oosterom R, Neufeld M, Del Pozo E (1985) The somatostatin analog SMS 201-995 induces long-acting inhibition of growth hormone secretion without rebound hypersecretion in acromegalic patients. J Clin Endocrinol Metab 60:1161

4. Lamberts SWJ, Uitterlinden P, Verleun T (1987) Relationship between growth hormone and somatomedin-C levels in untreated acromegaly, after surgery and radiotherapy and during medical therapy with sandostatin (SMS 201-995). Eur J Clin Invest 17:354

5. Lamberts SWJ, Uitterlinden P, Verschoor L, van Dongen KJ, Del Pozo E (1985) Long-term treatment of acromegaly with the somatosta-

tin analogue SMS 201-995. N Engl J Med
313:1576
6. Lamberts SWJ, Zweens M, Klijn JGM, Van
Vroonhoven CCJ, Stefanko SZ, Del Pozo E
(1986) The sensitivity of growth hormone and
prolactin secretion to the somatostatin analog
SMS 201-995 in patients with prolactinomas
and acromegaly. Clin Endocrinol 25:201

7. Lamberts SWJ, Zweens M, Verschoor L, Del
Pozo E (1986) A comparison among the
growth hormone-lowering effects in acromegaly of the somatostatin analog SMS 201-
995, bromocriptine, and the combination of
both drugs. J Clin Endocrinol Metab 63:16

25b. Sandostatin® (SMS 201-995) Can Exert a Direct Analgesic Effect

A. Beckers[1], A. Stevenaert[1], E. Bastings[1], M. de Longueville[2], G. Hennen[1]

[1] Endocrinologie, Neurochirurgie, Centre Hospitalier Universitaire, Liège, Belgium, and [2] Sandoz, Brussels, Belgium

We have been treating thirty acromegalic patients with Sandostatin® for 2 years. Sandostatin has proved to be very efficient in normalizing growth hormone (GH) and somatomedin-C (Sm-C) levels. Clinically, improvement began after two or three days of treatment. A decrease in soft tissue swelling was observed, paresthesias disappeared and headaches improved. In three cases, headaches disappeared entirely only a few minutes after Sandostatin injection. We should like to document these typical cases more precisely.

Patients, Methods and Results

Patient 1

This patient, a 34-year-old man, had been suffering for 3 years from severe headaches associated with a macroadenoma. He underwent unsuccessful transsphenoidal surgery and was subsequently treated by radiotherapy (4500 rads) with limited beneficial effects. The headaches, however, remained unaffected. Treatment with Sandostatin was thus initiated. The headaches disappeared entirely a few minutes after the first subcutaneous injection (50 µg) and reappeared after 6 hours. The same effect was obtained after each subcutaneous injection.

Surprisingly, long-term treatment with low doses of Sandostatin (6×50 µg/day subcutaneously) suppressed the headaches but was ineffective in normalizing GH and Sm-C levels, which remained at 15 ng/ml and 3 U/ml respectively. Headaches reappeared immediately upon cessation of treatment, as well as during placebo injections.

Higher doses of Sandostatin (6×100 µg/d) had the same effect on headaches but normalized GH and Sm-C levels and clinical signs of acromegaly.

Patient 2

This patient (33 years) had been suffering from severe headaches for 5 years. He had been operated upon in 1984 with clinical remission of acromegaly but without any effect on the headaches. Two years later, clinical signs of acromegaly reappeared (GH 5.6 ± 0.9 ng/ml; 12-h profile; Sm-C 3.6 U/ml) and the patient was treated with Sandostatin. As in case 1, headaches disappeared a few minutes after the first Sandostatin injection. Headaches and clinical signs of acromegaly disappeared entirely with prolonged treatment (GH 1.73 ± 1.1 ng/ml; 12-h profile, and Sm-C 0.4 U/ml after 2 months).

Patient 3

This later patient (34 years) presenting with active acromegaly (GH: 20 ng/ml) and severe headaches, did not receive any treatment prior to Sandostatin. The first injection had the same effects as in the two previous patients, and these effects were maintained during subsequent injections.

Conclusions

Recently, reviewing the effects of Sandostatin in man, Bloom and Polak [1] noted improvement of headaches in acromegaly, stating that this was unrelated to normalization of GH secretion.

Our results confirm that Sandostatin could act on headaches by mechanisms other than control of GH secretion or decrease of tumor size. Moreover, one single blind study excludes a placebo effect. Sandostatin can probably exert a strong and immediate analgesic effect by a way which remains to be explored and differs from that acting on GH control.

Reference

1. Bloom SR, Polak JM (1987) Somatostatin. Br Med J 295:288−290

25c. Relapsing Acromegaly Resistant to Both Bromocriptine and Sandostatin® Treatment

A. Beckers[1], A. Stevenaert[1], E. Bastings[1], M. de Longueville[2], G. Hennen[1]

[1] Endocrinologie, Neurochirurgie, Centre Hospitalier Universitaire, Liège, Belgium, and [2] Sandoz, Brussels, Belgium

Thirty acromegalic patients were treated in our hospital with Sandostatin® for a period of two years. The substance appeared effective in 70% of the cases. However, in some cases the effects were poor or nil. We describe here a patient whose acromegaly could be improved neither by surgery and radiotherapy nor with high doses of Sandostatin and bromocriptine.

Patient and Methods

The propositus, a 47-year-old man, had been operated upon in 1977 and reappeared in our clinic in 1985 with active acromegaly due to a large suprasellar extending tumor (stage IV according to Vezina and Maltais). He underwent transsphenoidal surgery but the fibrous tumor could not be resected and the patient thus received radiotherapy (4500 rads). This treatment did not improve clinical conditions. The patient received various forms of bromocriptine (Parlodel®[1] 20 mg daily per os and Parlodel LAR) without any added beneficial effect. He was then treated with increasing regimens of Sandostatin up to 3000 µg daily. The treatment failed to improve clinical conditions. We therefore tried intravenous administration. The test was performed as follows: subcutaneous injections of Sandostatin were stopped the day before the test at 22 h. The i.v. test began at 10 am with a starting rate of 1440 µg/24 h. Blood pressure was recorded as 170/110 mmHg and measurements of blood pressure were taken every 15 min. Blood samples were collected every 15 min for GH measurements. After one hour, the rate was increased twofold (2880 µg/24 h) but could not be prolonged because of elevation of blood pressure (20/11 mmHg). The rate was then reduced to the initial value (1440 µg/24 h) until 19 h until blood pressure returned to previous values. At 15 h, 5 mg Parlodel was given per os.

The treatment with 3000 µg subcutaneously was then reinstituted and complemented by intramuscular injection of Parlodel LAR.

A CT scan was performed before the beginning of Sandostatin treatment and one month after the injection of Parlodel LAR.

Results (Figs. 1, 2 and 3)

These treatments failed to achieve any clinical improvement although, biologically, a decrease of 50% in GH serum level and a slight decrease in Sm-C level were observed.

A further decrease was obtained when Parlodel LAR was administered simultaneously with Sandostatin.

The intravenous administration of Sandostatin resulted in decreased GH levels especially with the high rate regimen but failed to normalize GH secretion. Addition of oral bromocriptine resulted in a further slight decrease in GH level.

When Parlodel LAR was given to the patient, especially after the first injection, GH level was further reduced but remained abnormally high.

The CT scan revealed no change of tumor size.

No side effects were observed.

---

[1] Also marketed as Pravidel

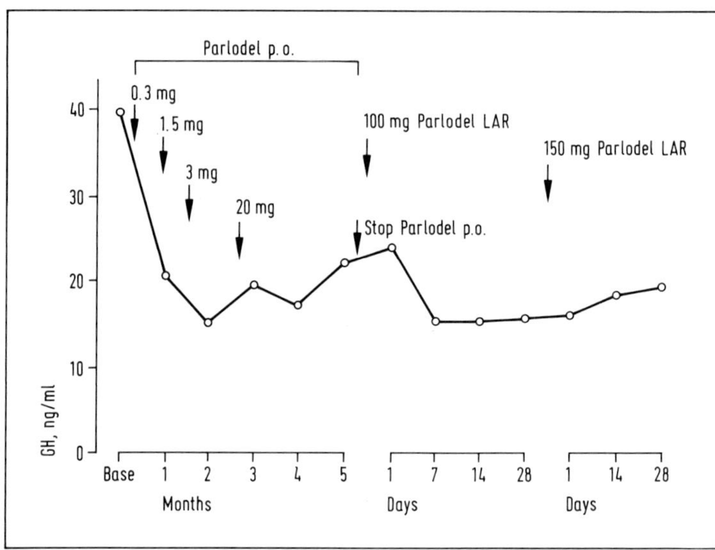

Fig. 1. Biological data (growth hormone, GH) during chronic treatment with Sandostatin and Parlodel

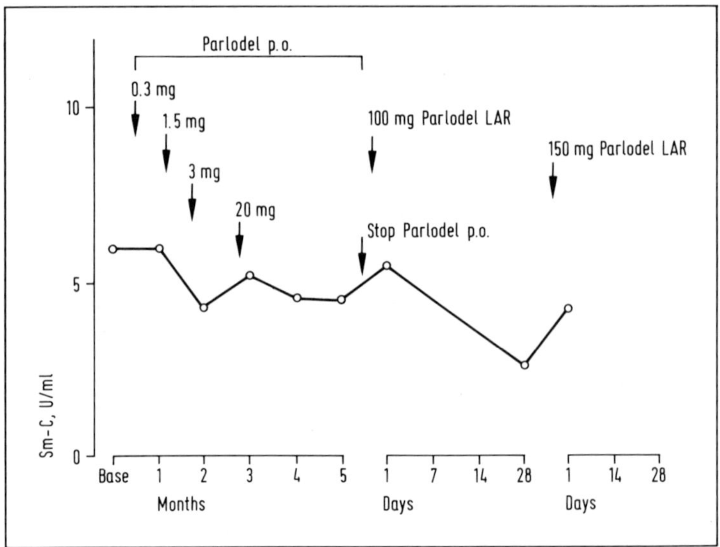

Fig. 2. Biological data (somatomedin-C, Sm-C) during chronic treatment with Sandostatin and Parlodel

Discussion

This case illustrates the difficulties encountered in the treatment of some acromegalic patients.

The treatment tried here had a slight lowering effect on biological parameters but remained ineffective on clinical signs and symptoms. Although high dosages of Sandostatin were used, they produced no side effects except when administered intravenously.

In the latter case, elevation of blood pressure is not necessarily related to intravenous Sandostatin administration.

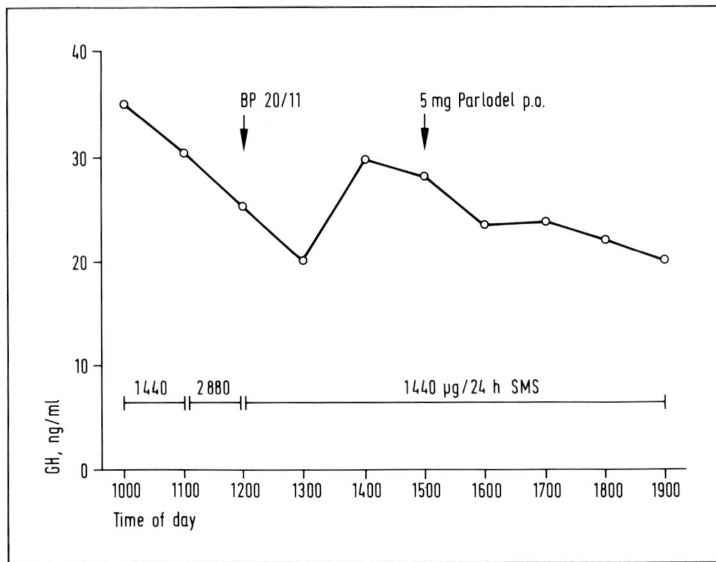

Fig. 3. Biological data (growth hormone, GH) during Sandostatin infusion

26. Consensus Discussion and Conclusions

J. Ginsburg

The Royal Free Hospital, London, UK

A consensus view of the role of Sandostatin® in acromegaly and the indications for its use were formulated after discussion of the various papers and posters presented at the meeting. For this purpose the participants separated into three working parties which reviewed Sandostatin therapy in (I) newly diagnosed and previously untreated acromegalic patients, in (II) treatment of the perioperative period before pituitary surgery or in (III) previously treated acromegalic patients where surgery and/or radiotherapy had failed to control activity of the acromegalic process. The reports of the working parties were then presented at a gathering of all participants and recommendations made to guide those using the drug for the first time. The ensuing discussion also highlighted the many aspects requiring further assessment and the difficulty of conducting a "conventional" drug trial in patients with acromegaly.

Test for Diagnosis of Acromegaly and Monitoring of Treatment

Diagnostic tests for acromegaly and for assessing effects of treatment on the progression of the disease had been discussed on several occasions during the meeting. Overall, it was agreed that if only one test was to be the hallmark for diagnosis in newly presenting patients, the favourite was somatomedin-C determination. The growth hormone response to an oral glucose tolerance test with suppression of growth hormone to below 2 ng/ml, the previous "gold standard", ran a close second. For optimal evaluation before deciding on therapy and in research studies, determination of the growth hormone profile over several hours was recommended. However, this is a tedious, time-consuming and labour-intensive test. Frequent sampling is essential; otherwise pulses and "spikes" of growth hormone activity are missed. Profile determinations are therefore not suitable for routine diagnostic use.

With current tests, there is also the problem of methodology. Results from different centres cannot therefore always be compared. The lack of uniformity in standards, as well as in different assay procedures, accounts for much of the variation. The possibility was discussed that industry might help ensure uniformity and homogeneity of assay methods by providing standards for this purpose.

Interpretation of test results and of the effects of therapy are further complicated by the lack of criteria for normality of certain parameters. Growth hormone secretion, for example, varies with age, stress, gonadal steroid concentration (in particular "free" estradiol levels) and with the state of nutrition (see Chapter 1). Thus, elevated levels may be found in malnourished subjects, as in anorexia nervosa. Similarly, fasting can increase growth hormone concentration within 18 h. Patients with diabetes mellitus and especially those with poor diabetic control, may also have markedly elevated growth hormone levels. Age, nutritional status and the presence of diabetes, renal or hepatic dysfunction must therefore be taken into account when assessing the significance of raised growth hormone concentrations. Furthermore, in view of the episodic nature of growth hormone secretion, frequent sampling over several hours may be required for accurate diagnosis. Somatomedin-C generation is also influenced by nutritional status and levels may be further influenced by concurrent drug intake such as estrogens.

The correlation between levels of growth hormone and somatomedin-C in different circumstances, was discussed by Stevenaert (see Chapter 13) and also by Lamberts (see Chapter 8), who have shown, in keeping with Lindholm et al. [11], that there is good correlation between plasma growth hormone and somatomedin-C concentrations in acromegalic patients after transsphenoidal hypophysectomy, *except* when plasma growth hormone concentrations are low. In these circumstances, patients regarded as "cured" on clinical grounds after surgery and in whom growth hormone levels were acceptably low by any criteria, may nevertheless show elevated somatomedin-C. And even patients with clinically active acromegaly may have low basal growth hormone concentrations, and also in response to oral glucose, but a significantly elevated somatomedin-C.

However, whilst a consensus view could be agreed on tests for diagnosing acromegaly, how to assess the effects of different types of treatment and define the criteria for normality after surgery or drug therapy was more difficult. No consensus was reached on the precise level of growth hormone which might be considered "ideal" after treatment of acromegaly or represent a "cure". A 50% reduction in growth hormone concentration, for example, might correlate well with marked clinical improvement after surgery or drug therapy but would certainly not be considered "normal" for a patient presenting de novo. Nevertheless, it was accepted that a single growth hormone estimation of less than 5 ng/l, as previously used, was inadequate for current purposes.

Similarly, no agreement was reached regarding interpretation of dynamic tests after surgery, such as oral glucose tolerance, the TRH test or growth hormone profiles.

Aims of Treatment and Recommended Schedules

The objectives of treatment in acromegaly are to suppress excess growth hormone secretion and to control or remove neoplastic growth whilst at the same time preserving and/or restoring normal pituitary function. These objectives are, however, rarely achieved with current surgical procedures or with radiotherapy. Furthermore, although the Sandostatin trials had shown that we could reverse the clinical abnormalities of acromegaly and restore normal endocrine function by treatment with this drug, we were still not able to "cure" the condition, for growth hormone hypersecretion recurred when drug therapy was discontinued.

Considerations other than biochemical normalization, the criteria for which, as discussed above, are in any event not absolute, may influence the precise type of treatment given to a new acromegalic patient as well as its timing. Thus, the clinical response of the patient is as important as the precise reduction achieved in growth hormone concentration. Preservation of pituitary function is particularly important for women who wish to conceive.

Microadenomas

Treatment schedules in patients with a microadenoma were considered separately from those with a large pituitary tumour. With the former, it was agreed that, providing an experienced neurosurgeon was available, the first line of treatment should be transsphenoidal pituitary surgery. If surgery failed, Sandostatin therapy should be initiated. If, however, there was persistent hyperprolactinaemia after surgery, then oral therapy with a dopamine agonist such as bromocriptine could be prescribed. If this proved ineffective, or was unacceptable because of side effects, then Sandostatin should be given. There was no contraindication to combined therapy with bromocriptine and Sandostatin, and indeed in a few patients there was some evidence of interaction between the two drugs and potentiation of bromocriptine activity by Sandostatin [9]. In view, however, of the hazards of radiotherapy (in particular the development of hypopituitarism) and the length of time before its effect on the progression of acromegaly became apparent, it was felt that radiotherapy should only be performed after weighing the relative hazards of this treatment and all other indications in individual patients. On the other hand, radiotherapy might be the treatment of choice in certain cases, e.g. those intolerant of oral drug therapy or where the costs of drug therapy were a major consideration.

Should Sandostatin be given before surgery to patients with a microadenoma? Pretreatment with the drug had been applied in some patients but, in view of the small number studied to date and the absence of controls for this purpose, no firm conclusion could yet be drawn as to any benefit of the drug in such cases. The precise indication for prescribing Sandostatin in the initial treatment of acromegaly associated with a pituitary microadenoma requires investigation. However, it was agreed that pretreatment with Sandostatin in such patients would not be detrimental.

Macroadenomas

A different schedule is proposed for treatment of large pituitary tumours. Mixed growth hormone and prolactin producing tumours may respond to a dopamine agonist such as bromocriptine. Combined Sandostatin and bromocriptine therapy was considered, in view of the fact that the clinical response to the latter might be limited and that some patients might be intolerant of bromocriptine. This also requires assessment in future trials. It was, however, accepted that patients presenting with large tumours not associated with hyperprolactinaemia, should have Sandostatin pretreatment. This apparently makes the tumours softer and subsequent surgery easier, an effect contrasting with the fibrosis observed after bromocriptine pretreatment of pure prolactin-producing tumours [10].

Several workers showed that preoperative use of Sandostatin in macroadenoma reduced tumour size but the speed and extent of this effect were not defined. Accurate definition of tumour size by CT scanning or MRI is therefore essential in future studies.

Successful treatment of visual field abnormalities and ophthalmic complications of pituitary tumours by Sandostatin has also been reported (see Chapters 22 and 23). Opinions were, however, divided as to whether Sandostatin should be the first line of treatment in such cases or whether pituitary surgery was the initial treatment of choice. Again, the availability of adequate neurosurgical skills is vital. In their absence or in an interim period, it was recommended that Sandostatin should be given.

Since tumour size in acromegaly is apparently negatively correlated with age [2], it was suggested that these neoplasms grew more rapidly in the young and that therapy should therefore be more aggressive in younger patients with acromegaly. A combination of surgery and intensive drug therapy should be considered in such cases.

The optimal duration of Sandostatin pretreatment before surgery has not yet been established. An arbitrary three months was proposed but trials are required to establish the degree of pituitary tumour shrinkage which might be induced by Sandostatin, together with the optimum dosage and duration of such therapy.

Clinical Effects

All those concerned with the study of Sandostatin commented favourably on the rapidity of clinical improvement after patients were started on Sandostatin and on the high proportion of responders. On average, only 10% of patients failed to respond clinically to Sandostatin treatment. In some series the response was as high as 87% (Fig. 1); the lowest response rate was 70% (see Chapter 13). Clinical improvement was generally observed very soon after starting therapy. Reduction in soft tissue swelling and excess perspiration, for example, was noted within two to four days of the start of treatment. Headache was also ameliorated in a high proportion and, indeed, in one patient with particularly severe headache, relief was obtained within minutes of the injection of Sandostatin. This effect raises the possibility of an analgesic action of the drug.

Tolerance to Sandostatin was not observed, even in patients treated for more than 3 years. Tachyphylaxis in respect of inhibition of growth hormone secretion or changes in insulin or blood glucose concen-

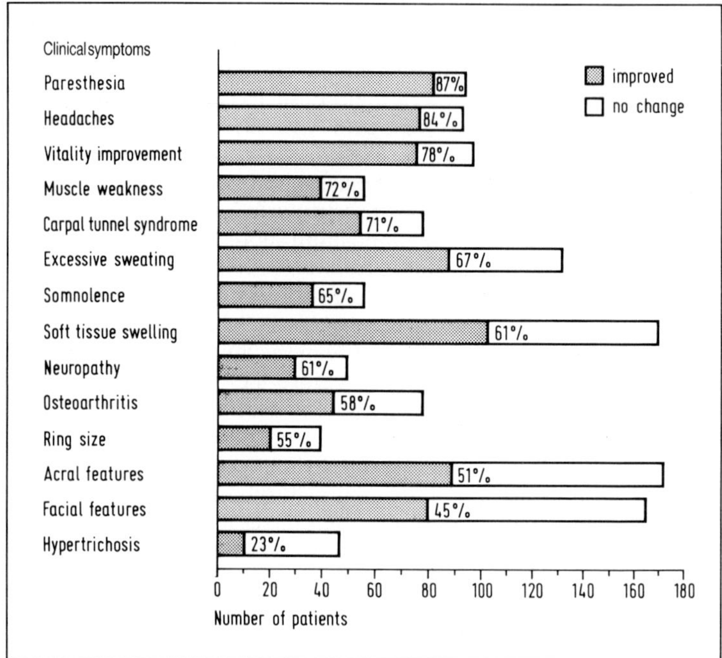

Fig. 1. Clinical improvement in acromegaly patients during treatment with Sandostatin. (Fig. 3 from Chapter 17, repeated here for convenience)

tration has not developed. After discontinuation of the drug, growth hormone levels rise and soft tissue changes gradually become apparent.

Side Effects

Sandostatin has relatively few side effects. The initial problem is that the injection itself may be painful. This can be minimized by warming the ampoule before withdrawing the solution and by giving the injection slowly. The pain is apparently due to the acetic acid component of the current diluent maintaining drug stability. The possibility was therefore raised that a different diluent might minimize injection pain.

The major side effects are gastrointestinal. Abdominal discomfort, nausea and diarrhea have been reported. These are generally only transient. The abdominal pain and nausea seem to be less or abolished if the Sandostatin is taken on an empty stomach. Diarrhea is accompanied, initially apparently, by increased fat excretion and thus seems to be a steatorrhea-like development. However, the increased fat content of the stools is only transient [6, 13]. Despite the relatively high incidence of loose stools at the start of treatment or when the dose was increased — 25 out of 40 patients in one series (see Chapter 12) — in only very few cases were the symptoms so severe as to necessitate stopping Sandostatin. Nausea and diarrhea are apparently less when the drug is given by continuous subcutaneous infusion. The claim (see Chapter 14) that administration of pancreatic enzymes relieves the diarrhea and abdominal pain was disputed.

Potentially, the most serious gastrointestinal effect seems to be gallstone formation. In a few cases, an apparently normal gall bladder ultrasound was present before starting treatment but asymptomatic gallstones were then observed after six months' Sandostatin. The precise incidence of new gallstone formation has not been established, since the initial trial protocol did not specify assessment of gall-bladder morphology *before* initiation of treatment. There seems to be some regional variation in incidence but whether this relates to dietary factors or the mode of drug administration is not known.

In future trials, accurate evaluation of gall-bladder morphology and function before starting treatment, and at intervals thereafter, are therefore required. Dietary habits must also be assessed before treatment. Some workers felt it was essential to perform a cholecystogram initially: ultrasound could give false positives and it was thought important to assess contractility of the organ in response to fat ingestion before and during treatment. It is not yet known whether the development of gallstones in patients taking Sandostatin can be prevented. Treatment of these gallstones is no different from that of asymptomatic calculi found in other situations.

Sandostatin, as expected, lowers circulating insulin levels. The insulin response to a carbohydrate meal is also attenuated (see Chapter 16). Nevertheless, there is no significant rise in fasting glucose or impairment of carbohydrate tolerance overall, presumably because of the fall in circulating growth hormone concentrations. The drug does not seem to exert a diabetogenic effect in the dosage given to control acromegaly. Indeed, there are reports of a fall in HbA_1C in diabetic patients (see Chapter 13). It is therefore possible, as demonstrated in monkeys (see Chapter 7) that the dose required for long-term inhibition of insulin release is considerably greater than that required for suppression of growth hormone in acromegalic subjects, which would make a long-acting preparation of Sandostatin particularly attractive.

Dosage and Mode of Administration

Sandostatin has been given in doses ranging from 150 that 3000 µg per day. It was, however, agreed that a t.d.s. regimen was required for, irrespective of the precise dose given, growth hormone concentration begins to rise after 5−7 h. A daily dose of 300 µg seems adequate for most patients, a conclusion reached initially from the results of a retrospective analysis of 178 cases (see Chapter 17) but corroborated by prospective studies currently totalling 62 patients (see Chapters 3, 11, and 12). Although patients have received stepwise increments of Sandostatin from 100 to 500 µg t.d.s., no greater benefit is apparent with the higher dosage.

It is of some interest, bearing in mind the considerable variation in sensitivity to Sandostatin in acromegalic subjects, that 100 µg t.d.s. seems adequate for the majority. The possibility has therefore been raised that the variation in sensitivity is related to receptor number and/or affinity as suggested by Reubi and Landolt [14].

Adjustment of dosage in those whose response to a standard dose of 100 µg Sandostatin t.d.s. is inadequate, can be assessed in relation to somatomedin-C concentration in the first instance. In view of the fact that pulsatility of growth hormone release continues, even in severe acromegaly, it was agreed that frequent sampling over several hours would be required for monitoring the growth hormone response to different doses of Sandostatin. This, as already mentioned, imposes a considerable workload on both doctor and patient. The minimum number of hours required for basal assessment or for determining the response to treatment was not, however, specified nor was the precise timing of samples, i.e. whether at 20-, 15- or 10-min intervals. Binding proteins can interfere with the assay and different laboratories, as already discussed, use different antibodies and standards.

Nevertheless, it was agreed that the dose of Sandostatin should be increased if the clinical response to the drug is inadequate. The problem is how long to wait before increasing the dose in different patients? No decision was taken as to whether this should be after one or after three months' treatment or even longer. It should be remembered that a further fall in somatomedin-C levels as well as clinical improvement have been observed after prolonged Sandostatin treatment at unchanged dosage [4].

Sandostatin had been given by continuous subcutaneous infusion using a transistorized infusion pump in some patients − a total dose of 100 to 600 µg over 24 h. Whereas with the t.d.s. regimen, there was a tendency for growth hormone concentration to rise shortly before each injection, hormone levels remained low throughout the 24 h during continuous subcutaneous infusion, even with a lower total dose. But whilst continuous infusion could give sustained drug levels and ensure continued suppression of growth hormone, this mode of administration is obviously not practicable for acromegalic patients receiving the drug on a chronic basis over months or years. Continuous drug infusion should be considered in selected cases over a limited period of time, e.g. patients with large tumours before surgery and where urgent decompression is required.

Pulsatile administration of Sandostatin with an initial dose of 10 μg every 2 h has been attempted (see Chapter 18a). The dose was increased, if necessary, up to 100 μg and the frequency similarly up to 16 times per 24 h. Whether pulsatile administration would give better control of growth hormone, particularly in those not responding to the recommended t.d.s regimen, is another aspect requiring future study.

Some workers thought it desirable to withdraw Sandostatin after a year's treatment so as to assess activity of the acromegalic process and decide whether any change in dosage was required. Unfortunately this counsel of perfection has proved difficult in practice, since patients generally felt so much better after starting on Sandostatin that they were extremely reluctant to discontinue treatment even for a few weeks.

Can the response to Sandostatin be predicted on the basis of changes in growth hormone over a few hours after administration of say 100 μg? No agreement was reached on this aspect despite the evidence presented in two recent papers [4, 12]. It was, however, emphasized that there was no reason to assume that Sandostatin acted solely on the pituitary and that it might have blocking actions elsewhere, e.g. the hypothalamus.

Although on first principles, it was agreed that Sandostatin should be discontinued if patients were found to be pregnant when taking the drug, there is as yet no information regarding the effects of Sandostatin in pregnancy.

Mechanism of Action of Sandostatin

The precise mechanism of action of the drug has not been determined, but it would seem that the initial effect is a decrease in growth hormone production. Studies of pituitary tumour cells in culture have shown a fall in growth hormone secretion within 24 h of Sandostatin administration. Thereafter, a significant decrease is also observed in the intracellular growth hormone content. It has therefore been suggested that tumour shrinkage after Sandostatin therapy reflects the combined effects of the inhibition in growth hormone secretion and the decreased size of tumour cells resulting from lowered intracellular growth hormone content [7]. A cytotoxic effect of the drug is unlikely since, when Sandostatin is withdrawn, growth hormone secretion resumes and elevated levels are found within a few days.

The mechanism whereby Sandostatin alters tumour cell consistency and induces liquefaction, which in itself may also affect tumour size, is not known. Similarly, the relation between responses to the drug and the histological nature of the tumour in different cases has not been assessed. If, therefore, a multicentre trial to establish the indications for preoperative use of Sandostatin is undertaken, it is essential that one centre is used for histological evaluation of tissue removed at surgery. The importance of including pituitary receptor studies in such trials was discussed. This raises a problem regarding the time of cessation of Sandostatin treatment prior to operation, since it is very difficult to carry out receptor studies in tissue where drug treatment has been continued right up to the time of surgery.

Unlike the natural hormone, somatostatin, withdrawal of the drug is not associated with any exaggerated rebound of growth hormone secretion.

Future Studies

To date, the majority of studies have been open trials. There is only one study of the acute effects of Sandostatin in acromegaly with placebo control [3, 8]. It should, however, be emphasized that because of the low prevalence of the condition (40/million [1]), multicentre trials are essential and a conventional double-blind placebo-controlled cross-over trial is not practicable. Moreover, the mounting evidence of the clinical and biochemical efficacy of the drug and of its superiority over other medical therapy for acromegaly, makes it unethical to deny patients effective treatment by giving them a placebo rather than Sandostatin.

Nevertheless, it was agreed that a number of questions had not been answered and several aspects needed careful evaluation in future trials. Assessment of gall-bladder motility and function before and after Sandostatin treatment, in association with investigation of the incidence of new gallstone formation after the drug, was thought to be an urgent matter for study. Other aspects which needed review included the long-term outcome of established and new diabetic acromegalic patients treated with Sandostatin; the length of pretreatment recommended before surgery and the dose required; long-term effects of the drug and the dose required for chronic therapy. The most important aspect calling for study was, however, the influence of Sandostatin on cardiovascular disease in acromegaly and, in particular, on the incidence of myocardial infarction and hypertension. Untreated acromegaly shortens life. Does Sandostatin influence life-expectancy? Does the drug affect morbidity and, if so, how?

Summary

Sandostatin is well tolerated and of low toxicity. The only side effects of the drug are transient gastrointestinal symptoms. Asymptomatic gallstone formation has been reported in a few cases but the precise incidence of this complication and the mechanism of gallstone formation after Sandostatin treatment are not known.

A marked and rapid clinical and biochemical improvement occurs after administration of the drug, headache being ameliorated within a matter of hours and a reduction in soft tissue swelling being apparent within two to four days. Circulating growth hormone concentrations fall within a few hours of Sandostatin administration.

The effects of the drug in acromegaly are reversible. Pretreatment levels of both growth hormone and somatomedin-C recur within days of stopping treatment but there is no rebound exaggerated secretion after discontinuation of therapy, as occurs with somatostatin. Tolerance to the drug has not

been observed even after three years' continuous treatment.

The current indications for Sandostatin treatment in acromegaly are:

1) patients in whom pituitary surgery or radiotherapy has failed to control the disease process;
2) patients unfit for surgery or unwilling to undergo pituitary surgery;
3) young patients concerned about fertility;
4) as an adjunct for softening macroadenoma and decreasing their size before pituitary surgery;
5) as an adjunct to radiotherapy in the interim period before the effects of radiotherapy on inhibition of growth hormone secretion are evident;
6) pretreatment with Sandostatin may also be considered in patients with acromegaly associated with a microadenoma although, provided adequate neurosurgical facilities are available, pituitary surgery should be untertaken in such cases.

A flow-chart showing the steps in the diagnosis of acromegaly and the appropriate therapeutic approaches is given in Figure 2.

The recommended starting dose is 100 µg t.d.s., s.c. In a few cases the drug has also been given by continuous subcutaneous infusion or in a pulsatile manner. The precise duration of treatment with Sandostatin and the optimal drug dosage for long-term therapy are still under investigation.

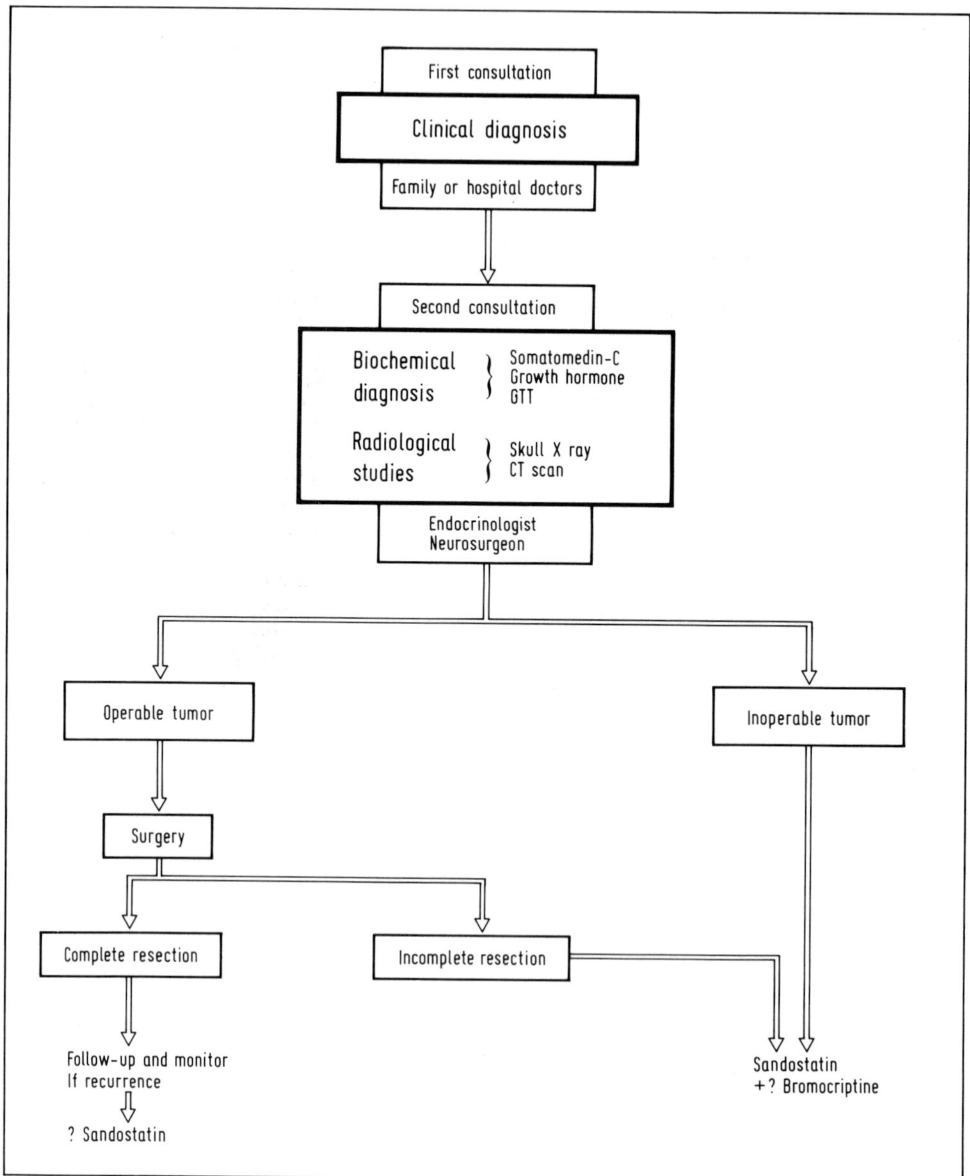

Fig. 2. Diagnosis and treatment of acromegaly

References

1. Alexander L, Appleton D, Hall R, Ross WM, Wilkinson R (1980) Epidemiology of Acromegaly in the Newcastle Region. Clin Endocrinol 12:71–79
2. Klijn JGM, Lamberts SWJ, de Jong FH, van Dongen KJ, Birkenhäger JC (1980) Inter-relationships between tumour size, age, plasma growth hormone and incidence of extrasellar extension in acromegalic patients. Acta Endocrinol 95:289–297
3. Lamberts SWJ, Oosterom R, Neufeld M, Del Pozo E (1985) The somatostatin analog SMS 201-995 induces long-acting inhibition of growth hormone secretion without rebound hypersecretion in acromegalic patients. J Clin Endocrinol Metab 60: 1161–1165

4. Lamberts SWJ, Uitterlinden P, Del Pozo E (1987) Sandostatin (SMS 201-995) induces a continuous further decline in circulating growth hormone and somatomedin-C levels during therapy of acromegalic patients for over two years. J Clin Endocrinol Metab 65:703−710

5. Lamberts SWJ, Uitterlinden P, Verleun T (1987) The relationship between growth hormone and somatomedin-C levels in untreated acromegaly, after surgery and radiotherapy and during medical therapy with Sandostatin (SMS 201-995). Eur J Clin Invest 17:354−359

6. Lamberts SWJ, Uitterlinden P, Verschoor L, van Dongen KJ, Del Pozo E (1985) Long-term treatment of acromegaly with the somatostatin analogue SMS 201-995. N Engl J Med 313:1576−1580

7. Lamberts SWJ, Verleun T, Hofland LJ, Del Pozo E (1987) A comparison between the effects of Sandostatin (SMS 201-995), bromocriptine and a combination of both drugs on hormone release by the cultured pituitary tumour cells of acromegalic patients. Clin Endocrinol (Oxf) 27:11−23

8. Lamberts SWJ, Zweens M, Klijn JGM, van Vroonhoven CCJ, Stefanko SZ, Del Pozo E (1986) The sensitivity of growth hormone and prolactin secretion of the somatostatin analogue SMS 201-995 in patients with prolactinomas and acromegaly. Clin Endocrinol (Oxf) 25:201−212

9. Lamberts SWJ, Zweens M, Verschoor L, Del Pozo E (1986) A comparison among the growth hormone-lowering effects in acromegaly of the somatostatin analog SMS 201-995, bromocriptine, and the combination of both drugs. J Clin Endocrinol Metab 63:16−19

10. Landolt AM, Keller PJ, Froesch ER, Müller J (1982) Bromocriptine: does it jeopardise the results of later surgery for prolactinomas? Lancet II:657−658

11. Lindholm J, Giwercman B, Giwercman A, Astrup J, Bjerre P, Skakkebaek NE (1987) Investigation of the criteria for assessing the outcome of treatment in acromegaly. Clin Endocrinol (Oxf) 27:553−562

12. Pieters GFFM, Smals AGH, Kloppenborg PWC (1986) Long-term treatment of acromegaly with the somatostatin analogue SMS 201-995. N Engl J Med 314:1391 (letter)

13. Plewe G, Schrezenmeir J, Nölken G, Krusse U, Beyer J, Kasper H, Del Pozo E (1986) Long-term treatment of acromegaly with the somatostatin analogue SMS 201-995 over 6 months. Klin Wochenschr 64:389−392

14. Reubi JC, Landolt AM (1984) High density of somatostatin receptors in pituitary tumors from acromegalic patients. J Clin Endocrinol 59:1148−1153